TOP FIVE
CAMPGROUNDS

BEST FOR SCENERY

1. 17 BUTTERFLY LAKE
2. 3 TONY GROVE
3. 15 TIMPOONEKE
4. 36 RED CLIFFS
5. 39 PINE LAKE

BEST FOR PRIVACY

1. 28 CLEAR CREEK
2. 38 HITTLE BOTTOM
3. 34 OAK GROVE
4. 19 BALSAM
5. 2 PIONEER

BEST FOR SPACIOUSNESS

1. 10 REDMAN
2. 17 BUTTERFLY LAKE
3. 33 CEDAR CANYON
4. 7 MONTE CRISTO
5. 26 MAPLE GROVE

BEST FOR QUIET

1. 37 LAVA POINT
2. 29 SIMPSON SPRINGS
3. 4 WILLARD BASIN
4. 28 CLEAR CREEK
5. 38 HITTLE BOTTOM

BEST FOR SECURITY

1. 4 WILLARD BASIN
2. 46 ELKHORN
3. 34 OAK GROVE
4. 37 LAVA POINT
5. 28 CLEAR CREEK

BEST FOR CLEANLINESS

1. 26 MAPLE GROVE
2. 50 GOBLIN VALLEY
3. 43 LONESOME BEAVER
4. 41 HAMBURGER ROCK
5. 35 SNOW CANYON

BEST FOR WHEELCHAIRS

1. 18 YELLOWPINE
2. 40 FRUITA
3. 14 ROCK CLIFF
4. 50 GOBLIN VALLEY
5. 35 SNOW CANYON

FAMILY-FRIENDLY

1. 50 GOBLIN VALLEY
2. 39 PINE LAKE
3. 14 ROCK CLIFF
4. 20 ASPEN GROVE
5. 1 ANTELOPE ISLAND

THE BEST IN TENT CAMPING

A GUIDE FOR CAR CAMPERS WHO HATE RVs, CONCRETE SLABS, AND LOUD PORTABLE STEREOS

UTAH

Jeffrey Steadman

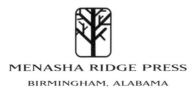

MENASHA RIDGE PRESS
BIRMINGHAM, ALABAMA

To Karen, whose patience fills these pages

 Printed on recycled paper

Library of Congress Cataloging-in-Publication Data

Steadman, Jeffrey.
   The best in tent camping : Utah : a guide for car campers who hate RVs,
   concrete slabs, and loud portable stereos / Jeffrey Steadman. —1st ed.
      p. cm.
   Includes bibliographical references and index.
      ISBN-13: 978-0-89732-647-6 (alk. paper)
      ISBN-10: 0-89732-647-4 (alk. paper)
   1. Camp sites, facilities, etc.—Utah—Directories. 2. Camping—Utah—Guidebooks.
   3. Utah—Guidebooks. I. Title.
      GV191.42.U8S74 2007
      796.5409792--dc22
      2007005334

Cover and text design by Ian Szymkowiak (Palace Press International)
Cover photograph by Taylor Kennedy/Alamy
Cartography by Jeffrey Steadman and Jennie Zehmer
Indexing by Jan Mucciarone

Menasha Ridge Press
P.O. Box 43673
Birmingham, Alabama 35243
www.menasharidge.com

TABLE OF CONTENTS

NORTHERN UTAH

WESTERN UTAH

SOUTHERN UTAH

APPENDIXES AND INDEX

ACKNOWLEDGMENTS

TO THE COUNTLESS CAMPGROUND HOSTS; Forest Service, Bureau of Land Management, and state park employees; and town locals for answering my odd questions, even if they were always accompanied by a raised eyebrow.

To everyone at Menasha Ridge for giving me the opportunity, motive, and excuse to go camping as much as possible.

To my father, Kerry, for introducing me to the outdoors. Without him, there is no book.

To my family—my mother, Robyn; sister, Jenn; and brothers Richy T. (I'll never get used to calling you that), Gergy, and Scottito-bandito. To Bob, Bev & Co.—Bob for the company in the backcountry, Bev & Co. for loaning me their Bob.

To my grandparents Fern and Blaine for taking care of my wife when I was gone to ensure I would still be married when I came home.

To the Eagle Boys of Midvale's Troop 400 for the once-a-month-no-matter-what campouts. Scotty, Jared, Tavin, Marcus, Zac, Job, Adam, Cory, Andy, and Mason: You are mighty badgers!

To Kate, Cecilia, and Dr. V for thinking I had skills enough to do something like this. I am writed good book!

To Aaron and the fellas at Wagco for keeping me solvent.

No animals were harmed in the making of this book. Unless you count the bird that I hit on Highway 12. But that was his fault—he totally flew into me.

PREFACE

U **TAH IS AWESOME.** From the highest snowcapped peaks in the north to the most colorful red rock canyon in the south, it is an amazing and inspiring place that you could spend a lifetime exploring.

Hopefully this book will serve as a launching pad into some of the best adventures the state has to offer. Who knows—within these pages might be a campground that becomes a family favorite, or the perfect place to stage a new hike you've been aching to try.

Fees get raised, campgrounds get renovated, and information changes about these campgrounds. Visit **www.jeffreysteadman.com** for all the up-to-date information including photographs of each campground. You can also report updates you've discovered and help other campers (and myself) stay informed.

People often ask me what my favorite campground is. Asking me to name my favorite campground is like asking a mother to pick her favorite child. It really depends on the day, my mood, and who's asking. I've seen places that I never imagined could exist. I've been to five national parks, a half dozen state parks, and through nearly every section of seven national forests. They're all so different, it would be impossible to compare them to select my favorite.

When I started this book, I really thought I would find an answer to that question. Instead, I've only found more questions. Like, "What's in the East Tintic Mountain Range," and "How long would it take me to hike from Survey Lake to the Grandaddy Lake Basin?" With every trip, my "To Do" list has gotten longer instead of shorter.

The campgrounds included here are the cream of the crop and will take you to spectacular locations. Each one holds something special that lifts it above the average campground. Your imagination and adventurous spirit will see with new eyes and maybe, just maybe, they'll inspire you to get outdoors a little more often.

In selecting the locations of these campsites, I've tried to balance the desire to be near some of Utah's best recreation opportunities with the ability to have a quality tent camping experience. For example, I've selected some incredible but lesser-known campgrounds just outside most of the national parks rather than right in the thick of the park. Exceptions to the rule are rare.

There are locations near the big cities—like Tanner's Flat and Botts Campgrounds and Snow Canyon State Park—that will help you realize how truly fortunate we are in Utah to have immediate access to the outdoors; and there are campgrounds like Clear Creek and Elkhorn that will open your eyes to the magnitude of the outdoors at your disposal. Both kinds are a treasure and a delight.

There's so much to see. So many great locations. So many ways to enjoy each one. The best thing you can do is just get in the car and start finding *your* questions.

I'll see you out there.

—Jeffrey Steadman

ABOUT THE AUTHOR

JEFFREY STEADMAN was born and raised in Utah, where he began exploring the outdoors shortly after leaving the womb.

As a child he spent his summertime exploring the canyons of the Wasatch Front on family hikes. In adulthood, the madness spread to winter, spring, and fall.

He's slept in snow caves, been in a hailstorm above the timberline at 12,000 feet, and once caught a fish out of a small stream on his birthday—with his bare hands. Usually he just uses a fishing pole. If all that 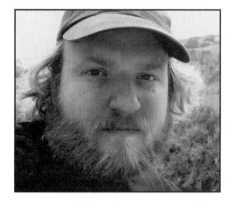 sounds a little gruff and grizzly, bear in mind he's also hosted a beauty pageant. More than once. And for more than one city.

When he's not in the backcountry, Jeffrey enjoys cooking, gardening, and acting. He and his wife, Karen, currently live in Midvale.

THE BEST
IN TENT
CAMPING
UTAH

THE BEST
IN TENT
CAMPING

UTAH

INTRODUCTION

WELCOME TO THE FIRST EDITION OF *The Best in Tent Camping: Utah.* If you're new to tent camping, or even if you're a seasoned camper, take a few minutes to read the following introduction. We explain how this book is organized and how to use it.

THE OVERVIEW MAP AND OVERVIEW-MAP KEY

Use the overview map on the inside front cover to assess the exact location of each campground. The campground's number appears not only on the overview map but also on the map key facing the overview map, in the table of contents, and on the profile's first page.

The book is organized by region as indicated in the table of contents. A map legend that details the symbols found on the campground layout maps appears on the inside back cover.

CAMPGROUND-LAYOUT MAPS

Each profile contains a detailed campground layout map that provides an overhead look at campground sites, internal roads, facilities, and other key items. Each campground entrance's GPS coordinates are included with each profile.

GPS CAMPGROUND-ENTRANCE COORDINATES

This book also includes the GPS coordinates for each campground entrance in two formats: latitude–longitude and UTM. Latitude and longitude coordinates tell you where you are by locating a point west (latitude) of the 0° meridian line that passes through Greenwich, England, and north or south of the 0° (longitude) line that belts the Earth, aka the equator.

Topographic maps show latitude and longitude as well as UTM grid lines. Known as UTM coordinates, the numbers index a specific point using a grid method. The survey datum used to arrive at the coordinates in this book is WGS84 (versus NAD27 or WGS83). For readers who own a GPS unit, whether handheld or onboard a vehicle, the latitude–longitude or UTM coordinates provided on the first page of each profile may be entered into the GPS unit. Just make sure your GPS unit is set to navigate using WGS84 datum. Now you can navigate directly to the campground.

That said, however, readers can easily find all campgrounds in this book by using the directions given and the campground layout map, which shows at least one major road leading into the area. But for those who enjoy using the latest GPS technology to navigate, the necessary data has been provided. A brief explanation of the UTM coordinates from Butterfly Lake (page 58) follows.

UTM Zone	12
Easting	511199
Northing	4507757

The UTM zone number 12 refers to one of the 60 vertical zones of the Universal Transverse Mercator (UTM) projection. Each zone is 6 degrees wide. The easting number 511199 indicates in meters how far east or west a point is from the central meridian of the zone. Increasing easting coordinates on a topo map or on your GPS screen indicate that you are moving east; decreasing easting coordinates indicate you are moving west. The northing number 4507757 references in meters how far you are from the equator. Above and below the equator, increasing northing coordinates indicate you are traveling north; decreasing northing coordinates indicate you are traveling south. To learn more about how to enhance your outdoor experiences with GPS technology, refer to *GPS Outdoors: A Practical Guide For Outdoor Enthusiasts* (Menasha Ridge Press).

THE CAMPGROUND PROFILE

In addition to maps, each profile contains a concise but informative narrative of the campground, as well as individual sites. This descriptive text is enhanced with at-a-glance ratings and information, GPS-based trailhead coordinates, and accurate driving directions that lead you from a major road to the parking area most convenient to the trailhead. On the first page of each profile is a ratings box.

THE RATING SYSTEM

This book includes a rating system for Utah's 50 best tent campgrounds. Six campground attributes—beauty, privacy, spaciousness, quiet, security, and cleanliness—are ranked using a five-star system. A low rating in one or two areas, especially privacy and spaciousness, was not necessarily grounds for exclusion from this book. In some cases, the nature of the terrain just doesn't allow for big, private sites, yet the campground still may be well worth a visit. This system should help you find what you are looking for.

BEAUTY In judging beauty, I took into account both what the general area has to offer as well as the campground. The most beautiful campgrounds have sites that you just don't want to leave and locations with easy access to breathtaking scenery.

PRIVACY Privacy is determined by how much your neighbors can pay attention to what you are doing and you to what they are doing. The best campgrounds have plenty of shielding (shrubs and trees) between adjoining sites, as well as staggered sites (that is, the entrance to the site across the road is not directly opposite yours).

SPACIOUSNESS While this category contributes to the amount of privacy you have, it refers mostly to how much space you have to move around in. The sites at some campgrounds are surprisingly large—to the point of overkill; others are incredibly small.

QUIET My evaluations were influenced to a great extent by the presence of RVs and the kinds of visitors a park tends to get (campgrounds near urban areas, for example, usually are a bit noisy, as are those that cater to families with children). I also considered the extent to which you could get away from the fray at a particular campground. You can expect some variation within my ratings based on whether you visit a campground during the week or on a weekend; on holiday weekends, all bets are off.

SECURITY With few exceptions, I found Utah campgrounds to be very safe and secure due largely to the presence of campground hosts and park rangers making the rounds.

CLEANLINESS My judgments were based on the presence and remnants of past campers around the campsite (trash, tent stakes, burned logs, etc.) and on the restroom facilities. I did take into account that primitive toilets tend to be a little less tidy than the modern facilities, although there seemed to me to be little reason for either to be a mess.

WEATHER

Nothing ruins a good camping trip faster than bad weather. Winter in northern Utah means that precious few campgrounds are even open. Southern Utah has more camping available throughout the winter months, but nights can still be frigid and the days drizzly.

Spring and fall are excellent times to see the lowest and driest campgrounds in the state. Both will provide excellent displays of nature's cycle of life—death and rebirth. Autumn is delayed into October and November in southern Utah, when giant cottonwoods along the small creeks light up in yellow hues. By March, the once-naked branches are slipping on their green leaves once again.

When the heat of summer comes, campers flock to the mountains for relief. Snow remains in some campgrounds until June or even July, so it's important to verify your campground has opened for the season. The weather changes rapidly above 7,000 feet in elevation; rain is quite common in the afternoon. Come prepared with adequate ponchos, rainflies, and plenty of extra socks.

FIRST-AID KIT

A typical first-aid kit may contain more items than you might think necessary. These are just the basics. Prepackaged kits in waterproof bags (Atwater Carey and Adventure Medical make a variety of kits) are available. As a preventive measure, take along sunscreen and insect repellent. Even though there are quite a few items listed here, they pack down into a small space:

Ace bandages or Spenco joint wraps

Adhesive bandages, such as Band-Aids

Antibiotic ointment (Neosporin or the generic equivalent)

Antiseptic or disinfectant, such as Betadine or hydrogen peroxide

Aspirin or acetaminophen

Benadryl or the generic equivalent, diphenhydramine (in case of allergic reactions)

Butterfly-closure bandages

Epinephrine in a prefilled syringe (for people known to have severe allergic reactions to such things as bee stings)

Gauze (one roll)

Gauze compress pads (six 4- x 4-inch pads)

Matches or pocket lighter

Moleskin/Spenco "Second Skin"

Waterproof first-aid tape

Whistle (it's more effective in signaling rescuers than your voice)

ANIMAL AND PLANT HAZARDS

TICKS   Ticks like to hang out in the brush that grows around campsites and along trails. Hot summer months seem to explode their numbers, but you should be tick-aware during all months of the year. Ticks, which are arthropods and not insects, need a host to feast on in order to reproduce. The ticks that light onto you will be very small, sometimes so tiny that you won't be able to spot them. Primarily of two varieties, deer ticks and dog ticks, both need a few hours of actual attachment before they can transmit any disease they may harbor. Ticks may settle in shoes, socks, or hats, and may take several hours to actually latch on. The best strategy is to visually check yourself a couple of times a day, especially if you've gone out for a walk in the woods. Ticks that haven't attached are easily removed, but not easily killed. If you pick off a tick in the woods, just toss it aside. If you find one on your body at camp, you may want to dispatch it (otherwise it may find you again). For ticks that have embedded, removal with tweezers is best.

RATTLESNAKE

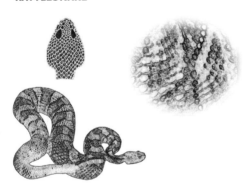

SNAKES   For the most part, snakes aren't a major concern for Utah campers. If you encounter a snake while camping or hiking, give it plenty of space and don't make any sudden movements. Most snakes aren't poisonous, but you don't ever want to test them to see for sure. Rattlesnakes do live in Utah (especially in more desert-like conditions), but I never saw one while researching this book.

POISON IVY/POISON OAK/POISON SUMAC   Recognizing poison ivy, oak, and sumac and avoiding contact with them is the most effective way to prevent the painful, itchy rashes associated with these plants. In the Southeast, poison ivy ranges from a thick, tree-hugging vine to a shaded ground cover, three leaflets to a leaf; poison oak occurs as either a vine or shrub, with three leaflets as well; and poison sumac flourishes in swampland, each leaf containing 7 to 13 leaflets. Urushiol, the oil in the sap of these plants, is responsible for the rash. Usually within 12 to 14 hours of exposure (but sometimes much later), raised lines and/or blisters will appear, accompanied by a terrible itch. Refrain from scratching because bacteria under fingernails can cause infection and you will spread the rash to other parts of your body. Wash and dry the rash thoroughly, applying a calamine lotion or other product to help dry the rash. If itching or blistering is severe, seek medical attention. Remember that oil-contaminated clothes, pets, or hiking gear can easily cause an irritating rash on you or someone else, so wash not only any exposed parts of your body but also clothes, gear, and pets.

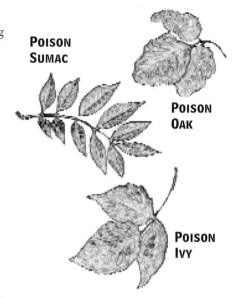

POISON SUMAC

POISON OAK

POISON IVY

MOSQUITOES Although it's not a common occurrence, individuals can become infected with the West Nile virus by being bitten by an infected mosquito. Culex mosquitoes, the primary varieties that can transmit West Nile virus to humans, thrive in urban rather than natural areas. They lay their eggs in stagnant water and can breed in any standing water that remains for more than five days. Most people infected with West Nile virus have no symptoms of illness, but some may become ill, usually 3 to 15 days after being bitten.

Late spring marks the beginning of the heavy mosquito season. In the high-elevation forests, you'll hear the buzzing swarms before you see them. Their numbers wane after the first good frost, but you can find them in every season but winter.

Utah officials have recommended using a repellent that contains Deet as its active ingredient. Deet has been used for more than 60 years and has proven to be safe and effective.

TIPS FOR A HAPPY CAMPING TRIP

There is nothing worse than a bad camping trip, especially since it is so easy to have a great time. To assist with making your outing a happy one, here are some pointers.

- Wherever possible, reserve your site ahead of time, especially if it's a weekend, a holiday, or if the campground is wildly popular. Many prime campgrounds require at least a six-month lead time on reservations. Check before you go.

- Pick your camping buddies wisely. A family trip is pretty straightforward, but you may want to consider including grumpy Uncle Fred who does not like bugs, sunshine, or marshmallows. After you know who is going, make sure that everyone is on the same page regarding expectations of difficulty, sleeping arrangements, and food requirements.

- Don't duplicate equipment such as cooking pots and lanterns among campers in your party. Carry what you need to have a good time, but don't turn the trip into a major moving experience.

- Dress appropriately for the season. Educate yourself on the highs and lows of the specific area you plan to visit. It may be warm at night in the summer in your backyard, but up in the mountains it will be quite chilly.

- Pitch your tent on a level surface—preferably one that is covered with leaves, pine straw, or grass—on a tarp or specially designed footprint to thwart ground moisture and to protect the tent floor. Do a little site maintenance such as picking up small rocks and sticks that can damage your tent floor and make sleep uncomfortable. If you have a separate tent rainfly but don't need it, keep it rolled up at the base of the tent in case it starts raining at midnight.

- If you are not used to sleeping on the ground, take a sleeping pad with you. Take one that is full-length and thicker than you think you might need. This will not only keep your hips from aching on hard ground, but will also help keep you warm.

- If you are not hiking in to a primitive campsite, there is no real need to skimp on food due to weight. Plan tasty meals and bring everything you will need to prepare, cook, eat, and clean up the mess.

- If you're prone to using the bathroom multiple times at night, you should plan ahead. Leaving a warm sleeping bag and stumbling around in the dark to find the restroom, whether it be an outhouse, a fully plumbed facility, or just the woods, is no fun if you're not sure where you're headed. Keep a flashlight and any other accoutrements you may need by the tent door and know exactly where to head in the dark. For guys, a practical (but often scoffed at) solution is to keep a large-mouth Nalgene-type bottle in the tent and use that inside the sleeping bag at night. Be discreet, though, and dispose of the night's work appropriately.

- Standing dead trees and storm-damaged living trees can pose a real hazard to tent campers. These trees may have loose or broken limbs that could fall at any time. When choosing a spot to rest or a backcountry campsite, look up.

CAMPING ETIQUETTE

Camping experiences can vary wildly depending on a variety of factors such as weather, preparedness, fellow campers, and time of year. Here are a few tips on how to create good vibes with fellow campers and wildlife you encounter.

- Obtain all permits and authorization as required. Make sure you check in, pay your fee, and mark your site as directed. Don't make the mistake of grabbing a seemingly empty site that looks more appealing than your site. It could be reserved. If you are unhappy with the site you've selected, check with the campground host for other options.

- Leave only footprints. Be sensitive to the ground beneath you. Be sure to place all garbage in designated receptacles or pack it out if none are available. No one likes to see the trash someone else has left behind.

- Never spook animals. It's common for animals to wander through campsites, where they may be accustomed to the presence of humans (and our food). An unannounced approach, a sudden movement, or a loud noise startles most animals. A surprised animal can be dangerous to you, to others, and to themselves. Give them plenty of space.

- Plan ahead. Know your equipment, your ability, and the area in which you are camping—and prepare accordingly. Be self-sufficient at all times; carry necessary supplies for changes in weather or other conditions. A well-executed trip is a satisfaction to you and to others.

- Be courteous to other campers, hikers, bikers, and others you encounter. Remember that they're probably out there to enjoy themselves just like you are.

- Strictly follow the campground's rules regarding the building of fires. Never burn trash. Trash smoke smells horrible and trash debris in a fire pit or grill is unsightly.

BACKCOUNTRY CAMPING ADVICE

A permit is usually not required before entering the backcountry to camp, but you should always check regulations before every backcountry trip. Take care to practice low-impact camping. Adhere to the adages "Pack it in, pack it out," and "Take only pictures, leave only footprints." Practice "Leave no trace" camping ethics while in the backcountry.

Check the latest regulations regarding campfires. Backpacking stoves are strongly encouraged. Admire the wildlife from a distance, because close interaction rarely ends well. When wildlife learns to associate backpacks and backpackers with easy food sources, their behavior may be changed forever. If you're in bear country, make sure you have about 40 feet of thin but sturdy rope to properly secure your food. Bear canisters are becoming increasingly popular and make bear-proofing your food a breeze. Ideally, you should throw your rope over a stout limb that extends ten or more feet above ground. Make sure the rope hangs at least five feet away from the tree trunk.

Solid human waste must be buried in a hole at least three inches deep and at least 200 feet away from trails and water sources; a trowel is basic backpacking equipment.

Following the above guidelines will increase your chances for a pleasant, safe, and low-impact interaction with nature.

VENTURING AWAY FROM THE CAMPGROUND

If you go for a hike, bike, or other excursion into the boondocks, here are some tips.

- **Always carry food and water** whether you are planning to go overnight or not. Food will give you energy, help keep you warm, and sustain you in an emergency situation until help arrives. You never know if you will have a stream nearby when you become thirsty. Bring potable water or treat water before drinking it from a stream. Boil or filter all found water before drinking it.

- **Stay on designated trails.** Most hikers get lost when they leave the path. Even on the most clearly marked trails, there is usually a point where you have to stop and consider which direction to head. If you become disoriented, don't panic. As soon as you think you may be off track, stop, assess your current direction, and then retrace your steps back to the point where you went awry. If you become absolutely unsure of how to continue, return to your vehicle the way you came in. Should you become completely lost and have no idea of how to return to the trailhead, remaining in place along the trail and waiting for help is most often the best option for adults and always the best option for children.

- **Be especially careful when crossing streams.** Whether you are fording the stream or crossing on a log, make every step count. If you have any doubt about maintaining your balance on a foot log, go ahead and ford the stream instead. When fording a stream, use a trekking pole or stout stick for balance and face upstream as you cross. If a stream seems too deep to ford, turn back. Whatever is on the other side is not worth risking your life.

- **Be careful at overlooks.** While these areas may provide spectacular views, they are potentially hazardous. Stay back from the edge of outcrops and be absolutely sure of your footing; a misstep can mean a nasty and possibly fatal fall.

- **Know the symptoms of hypothermia.** Shivering and forgetfulness are the two most common indicators of this insipid killer. Hypothermia can occur at any elevation, even in the summer, especially when the hiker is wearing lightweight cotton clothing. If symptoms arise, get the victim shelter, hot liquids, and dry clothes or a dry sleeping bag.

- **Take along your brain.** A cool, calculating mind is the single most important piece of equipment you'll ever need on the trail. Think before you act. Watch your step. Plan ahead. Avoiding accidents before they happen is the best recipe for a rewarding and relaxing hike.

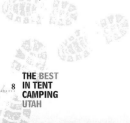

NORTHERN UTAH

1
ANTELOPE ISLAND STATE PARK

ANTELOPE **I**SLAND **IS STEEPED** in history. From Native Americans to ranchers, the Great Salt Lake's biggest island has a fascinating story. Stay at the Bridger Bay campground on the northwestern tip of the island and you can experience firsthand what this skinny island has to offer.

Evidence of Fremont Indians on Antelope Island pins their visits from 500 to 2,000 years ago, although archaeologists recently found a Humboldt-style arrowhead that could date back as far as 6,000 years. Modern settlement began here in 1848 when Fielding Garr moved to the island with his six children. The island became range for cattle, used to fund the Perpetual Emmigration Fund (a revolving loan account that funded immigration to Utah for early church converts) of the Church of Jesus Christ of Latter-Day Saints. Prominent citizens of early Utah, like Brigham Young, also kept their animals on the island. In 1875 the LDS church gave up control of the island and much of the property went to Union Pacific Railroad, homesteaders, and miners. Eventually land ownership consolidated into the Island Improvement Company, a corporate ranching enterprise that shifted ranching activities from cattle to sheep. In 1972 the island was sold to another ranching group. Nine years later, in 1981, Utah Parks and Recreation purchased the island and converted it to its present-day status as Antelope Island State Park.

There are two campgrounds on the island, and unfortunately neither is outrageously spectacular standing on its own merits. Still, telling your friends you spent the weekend camped on an island makes for a great story, so this is definitely a pretty cool camp destination.

Bridger Bay is the individual-use campground with 26 sites, most of which are pull-through. It's true that this campground will attract more hefty RVs, but Antelope Island isn't the kind of place where you typically

> *From Native Americans to ranchers, the Great Salt Lake's biggest island has a fascinating story.*

RATINGS

Beauty: ✿ ✿ ✿ ✿
Privacy: ✿ ✿
Spaciousness: ✿ ✿ ✿
Quiet: ✿ ✿ ✿ ✿
Security: ✿ ✿ ✿ ✿ ✿
Cleanliness: ✿ ✿ ✿ ✿

ADDRESS:	Antelope Island State Park 4528 West 1700 South Syracuse, UT 84075-6868
OPERATED BY:	Utah State Parks and Recreation
INFORMATION:	www.stateparks .utah.gov
OPEN:	Year-round
SITES:	26 (plus 12 nearby group sites)
EACH SITE HAS:	Picnic table, fire ring
ASSIGNMENT:	By reservation; first come, first served if available
REGISTRATION:	Online at www .reserveamerica.com; large groups call (801) 773-2941
FACILITIES:	Vault toilets, garbage service, drinking water, showers (except in winter), visitor center
PARKING:	At campsite only
FEE:	$12 per night, $9 park entrance
ELEVATION:	4,260 feet
RESTRICTIONS:	*Fires:* In rings only *Other:* 14-day stay limit

worry about raucous parties and wild campers. Instead, you'll find that most of the visitors here are fascinated by the interesting atmosphere created by the island.

The sites at Bridger Bay are spread around a large one-way loop. There's no vegetation taller than sagebrush, so you're just going to have to do without shade or shield from neighbors. Each plot has ample space to put a tent on the grassy ground by the table. Whiterocks Campground, found around the jutted land of Buffalo Point, is a group site. You may want to check it out (especially site 1) if you're dead set against staying close to other campers. The group sites are more spread out from each other, although the ground is only dirt and there's even less vegetation.

Antelope Island is heaven for a birder. The Great Salt Lake supports between two million and five million shore birds—two-thirds of all migratory waterfowl in North America—and is one of the top ten winter populations of bald eagles in the lower United States. Everything from avocets to white-faced ibis call this massive terminal basin home. If you're a hard-core birder, check out the Bear River Migratory Bird Refuge on the lake's northeastern tip, accessed back on the mainland by going north on Interstate 15 and then west on Bird Refuge Road at Brigham City. They've recently renovated the facility and have every resource available to help you learn about the birds in this globally important body of water.

You don't have to leave the island to see spectacular wildlife, though. And that's really the point of coming to stay at Bridger Bay: you've got wildlife all around you. You're sure to spot the common pasty white biped (aka humans) swimming in the Great Salt Lake. As a native Utahn, I take for granted the once-in-a-lifetime experience it is to test the unbelievable buoyancy of the salty water. I usually try to stay out of the stink, but you've got to try it at least once, and staying at the campground gives you the perfect excuse. You've got showers and sand about a mile away on a state-maintained beach. The stink is all in your head—swimming is actually a hoot!

Chase down more desirable wildlife encounters by heading back toward the visitor center and then turning

MAP

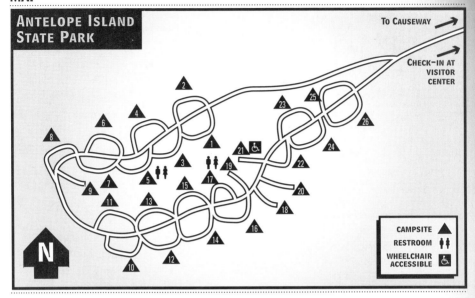

ANTELOPE ISLAND STATE PARK

To CAUSEWAY

CHECK-IN AT VISITOR CENTER

CAMPSITE	▲
RESTROOM	♟
WHEELCHAIR ACCESSIBLE	♿

N

right toward Buffalo Point. You'll follow the signs to the buffalo pens and see some of the meanest-looking animals around. About 600 head of buffalo roam the island, so take the long road around the southeastern side of the island to historic Fielding Garr Ranch and you should see at least one buffalo in a more natural environment. True to the song, deer and antelope play here too, along with bighorn sheep and coyote.

Fielding Garr Ranch has been preserved as a living museum, so walk the grounds and tour the different structures. The grounds are maintained by a caring staff, and large cottonwoods dot the area to provide shade on an otherwise exposed landscape. It's a perfect place to plop down for lunch. You'll also appreciate the comforts of your own home after seeing the not-so-cushy living quarters of the ranch home. Take the time to read the in-depth description of the island's heritage and you'll appreciate even more how special this place is.

Fall and spring are the best times to visit Antelope Island State Park. Even winter is preferable to the scorching heat in the summer. The bugs also kick into high gear when temperatures warm, so plan to come here when temperatures are still mild.

GETTING THERE

Take Interstate 15 Exit 332 west through Syracuse and across the 7.5-mile causeway to Antelope Island. Follow the signs to the campground.

GPS COORDINATES

UTM Zone: 12
Easting: 444910
Northing: 4569748
Latitude: N 41.27729
Longitude: W 111.65780

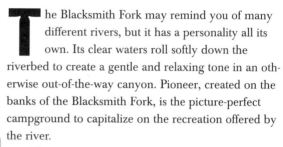

> *The Blacksmith Fork is in an elite class of Utah rivers known as Blue Ribbon Fisheries.*

The Blacksmith Fork may remind you of many different rivers, but it has a personality all its own. Its clear waters roll softly down the riverbed to create a gentle and relaxing tone in an otherwise out-of-the-way canyon. Pioneer, created on the banks of the Blacksmith Fork, is the picture-perfect campground to capitalize on the recreation offered by the river.

There are two sections of the campground, with the majority of the sites located on the main loop away from the road. After site 2, a funny little spur takes off to the right and leads to sites 3, 4, and 5. The best is site 3. It backs up into nothing but vegetation; sites 4 and 5 share boundaries with campsites along the main road. On the other fork of the road, found between sites 1 and 2, are 16 through 18. They are far removed from the main camp area, so if you're trying to get three sites together for a larger group, this setup is perfect. If it's just you, take site 17 for its distance from the others and its position right on the Blacksmith Fork river.

The Blacksmith Fork is in an elite class of Utah rivers known as Blue Ribbon Fisheries. This program, created in 2001, identified rivers and lakes that offered "quality angling experiences in aesthetically pleasing settings where the waters are environmentally productive and sustain healthy fish populations." Waters were selected on five criteria: water quality and quantity, accessibility, natural reproduction capability, angling pressure, and the presence of certain species.

Blacksmith Fork was an obvious selection. The 16-mile stretch from the first impoundment to Hardware Ranch excels in each of the criteria, and at Pioneer you're right in the thick of things. The river is known for its large, lumbering turns and gentle riffles. Keep an eye out for private property; about 28 percent of it falls into

RATINGS

Beauty: ☆ ☆ ☆ ☆
Privacy: ☆ ☆ ☆ ☆
Spaciousness: ☆ ☆ ☆
Quiet: ☆ ☆ ☆ ☆
Security: ☆ ☆ ☆
Cleanliness: ☆ ☆ ☆ ☆

that category. Mostly brown trout swim these waters, so nymphing and streamers seem to be most productive. Bait fishing is currently allowed on the river, so even the most impatient 6-year-old can have a shot at a brown, or even the occasional cutthroat or mountain whitefish.

Recent overabundance of brown trout has put forage at a minimum, and anglers have been encouraged to harvest more browns to thin the herd. Check the current fishing proclamation, as biologists are always monitoring the water, and conditions can quickly swing the other way.

If the main river is too crowded, try a detour up the Left Hand Fork. Forest Service Road 055 will take you to some areas with good public access. This is also a good backup plan if Pioneer is full—there are a couple of places to camp along the road.

Pig lovers are in hog heaven (pun intended) up FS 055. Just east of Spring Campground is the trailhead access for a hike to Hog Hole, Pig Hole, Boar Hole, and Sow Hole. I'm not really sure how large of a crowd that is—pig lovers, I mean—but this little loop hike to some of the area's pork-centric springs is bound to delight everyone down to the most dedicated vegetarian.

Just 7 miles east of camp is Hardware Ranch. While the name of the ranch may conjure up images of wild screwdrivers roaming the plains, and free-range nuts and bolts grazing in a meadow, the only creatures on display here are elk. The state of Utah purchased the ranch in 1945 from the Box Elder Hardware Company and established it as a place to study and manage the local elk herds, especially in winter months.

Elk have historically come down Blacksmith Fork Canyon into Cache Valley to feed during the winter, but by the early 20th century, homes and farms were starting to squeeze them out. Hardware Ranch was set up as a winter range for the elk, and each year the state grows tons of grass hay for the foraging herds. By their own recognition, natural range in Cache Valley would be ideal, but is simply impractical.

If you're staying at Pioneer, that probably means it's still relatively warm outside and the 500 to 600 elk that frequent the ranch haven't yet taken up residence. Still, drop in to the visitor center to learn more about elk

KEY INFORMATION

ADDRESS:	Wasatch-Cache National Forest Logan Ranger District 1500 East US 89 Logan, UT 84321
OPERATED BY:	Scenic Canyons
INFORMATION:	(435) 755-3620; www.fs.fed.us/r4/wcnf/unit/logan
OPEN:	May–September
SITES:	18
EACH SITE HAS:	Picnic table, fire pit
ASSIGNMENT:	First come, first served
REGISTRATION:	Self-register on-site
FACILITIES:	Vault toilets, drinking water, garbage service
PARKING:	At campsite only
FEE:	$13 per night, $6 extra vehicle
ELEVATION:	5,086 feet
RESTRICTIONS:	*Pets:* Leashed *Other:* 8 people per site

MAP

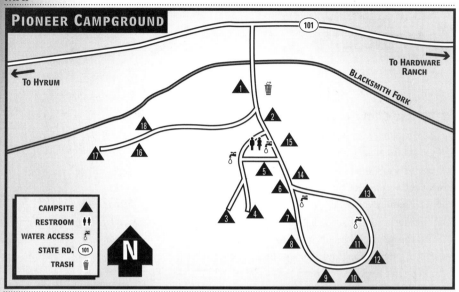

GETTING THERE

From Hyrum, go 9 miles east on UT 101.

and other wildlife near the ranch through interactive displays and staff programs. Mark your calendar for the annual fall Elk Festival and check into the sleigh rides offered each winter through the elk feeding grounds.

GPS COORDINATES

UTM Zone: 12
Easting: 442303
Northing: 4608805
Latitude: N 41.62889
Longitude: W 111.69266

3
TONY GROVE CAMPGROUND

TONY GROVE IS THE ALL-AMERICAN campground. This sizable but tidy location has it all: a lake nearby full of lively little fish, entrance to a fantastic trail system that leads to lakes and wilderness, easy access, and great campsites with plenty of room to set out your stuff.

Set deep into Wasatch-Cache National Forest off US 89, this perfect little playground at 8,000 feet does everything right. You'll wander up the Logan Canyon Scenic Byway and turn off onto Forest Service Road 003. As the road weaves its way up to Tony Grove, you pass through the lower canyon brush, then stands of aspens that finally give way to spruce, pine, and fir. The drive alone is enough to make the trip worth it, destination notwithstanding.

Don't misunderstand—here it's about the journey *and* the destination. As FS 003 ends, it gently delivers drivers into the small valley where Tony Grove Lake is located. At 25 acres, the lake is big enough to host more than a couple of canoes, but not yet big enough to be intimidating.

The campground is located on the lake's southeastern shore, accessed by following the short driveway from FS 003. For the most part, the campground is a large loop with a small tail at the entrance. Stay on the backside of the loop—sites 10 through 23ish—if you want to avoid a lot of foot traffic. Site 13 is off on its own, but you must climb a small stairway to reach it; arthritis sufferers beware. Sites 29 through 31 offer best access to the lake, although human nature indicates that you may have people traipsing through your campsite on their way to and from the lake. After the turn, sites 32 through 37 are perched somewhat on a hill but are still accessible.

Sites here are generally well spaced and well proportioned. The extra space helps numb that part of your

> *A good hike, a little fishing, a great campsite—what more could you ask for?*

RATINGS

Beauty: ☆ ☆ ☆ ☆ ☆
Privacy: ☆ ☆ ☆ ☆
Spaciousness: ☆ ☆ ☆ ☆ ☆
Quiet: ☆ ☆ ☆
Security: ☆ ☆ ☆ ☆
Cleanliness: ☆ ☆ ☆ ☆

ADDRESS:	Wasatch-Cache National Forest Logan Ranger District 1500 East US 89 Logan, UT 84321
OPERATED BY:	Scenic Canyons
INFORMATION:	(435) 755-3620; www.fs.fed.us/r4/ wcnf
OPEN:	July–October
SITES:	37
EACH SITE HAS:	Picnic table, fire pit
ASSIGNMENT:	First come, first served; reservations accepted
REGISTRATION:	Self-register on-site for available sites; reserve online at www.reserveusa.com or call (877) 444-6777
FACILITIES:	Vault toilets, drinking water, garbage service
PARKING:	At campsite only, $3 per day, $10 per week, $25 per season for non-campers
FEE:	$15 per night, $6 extra vehicle
ELEVATION:	8,037 feet
RESTRICTIONS:	*Pets:* Leashed *Other:* 7-day stay limit; 8 people per site

brain that acknowledges that the campground is almost always full. You won't forget that fact, but you certainly won't feel like you're camped next to 200 strangers. Because of high demand, many sites can be reserved. If you plan on showing up later than noon on a weekend, you'd best book ahead of time. If not, you're rolling the dice with the 23 first-come, first-served sites.

Bring your hiking boots to Tony Grove and try the White Pine Lake hike. It's a modest 1,250-foot elevation gain over a 3.5-mile (one-way) trip and ends at the lovely White Pine Lake between Mounts Gog and Magog, less than a half mile from the Mount Naomi Wilderness boundary. The main parking lot also hosts the trailhead to Naomi Peak itself. This trail requires a little more exertion out of its hikers, summiting just below 10,000 feet. Try to plan your hike in late July or early August and this hike will offer you a feast of wildflower colors on an alpine platter. You'll also be rewarded with views of several deep canyons that claw their way toward the peak in a sensational and sometimes eerily shadowed fashion.

Longer hikes to Green Canyon and High Creek actually funnel out to Cache Valley on the other side of the mountain. Hiked in reverse, this would be a great alternative to taking the paved roads to Tony Grove. Let a lesser outdoorsman take the car—you can hike the 10 or 15 miles from Cache Valley!

If you happen to be the lesser outdoorsman (or if you're just not crazy) take one of the shorter hikes. There's an interpretive nature trail near the lake that's made especially for sauntering.

Pack your fishing pole and try the action at Tony Grove Lake. It's stocked regularly, so you probably won't pull a record out of the water, but you've got a decent chance at catching your dinner. The Logan River is also a highly prized fishery, and anywhere along US 89 should yield a day of challenging but memorable fishing. Other small creeks in the area are hit-and-miss, but those can sometimes be the most rewarding experiences: miss … miss … hit!

If you've got a canoe, kayak, raft, or even inner tube, this is the place to bring it. Tony Grove Lake's frigid waters take some getting used to, but a quick

MAP

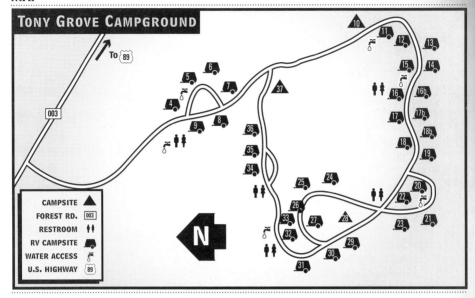

TONY GROVE CAMPGROUND

To 89

CAMPSITE	▲
FOREST RD.	003
RESTROOM	♦♦
RV CAMPSITE	🚐
WATER ACCESS	⌇
U.S. HIGHWAY	89

N

dunk in the water is just what the doctor ordered on a sunny summer afternoon. Paddle across the lake to get a better view of the cliffs that seem to hover over the lake as bodyguards.

It's a shame that Tony Grove is only open for a few months each summer. The snowmobiling crowd is fond of it in the winter, but it's just not the same. A good hike, a little fishing, a great campsite—what more could you ask for?

GETTING THERE

From Logan, go 22 miles east on US 89 and turn left on FS 003. Go 7 miles to the campground.

GPS COORDINATES

UTM Zone: 12

Easting: 446918

Northing: 4638192

Latitude: N 41.89388

Longitude: W 111.63989

4
WILLARD BASIN
CAMPGROUND

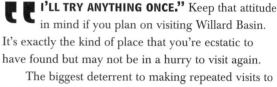

> *The basin calls to mind images of terraced rice paddies in Asia.*

"I'LL TRY ANYTHING ONCE." Keep that attitude in mind if you plan on visiting Willard Basin. It's exactly the kind of place that you're ecstatic to have found but may not be in a hurry to visit again.

The biggest deterrent to making repeated visits to Willard Basin is the car ride into the campground. Getting there is no picnic. For starters, the Willard Peak Scenic Byway isn't really labeled as such in town, so it's easy to lose your way. In Mantua, head south on Main Street, which becomes Willard Peak Road. You'll pass the large LDS church and continue on Willard Peak Road, which soon turns from pavement to dirt as it starts a slow ascent of the canyon. You'll find out fast that this road requires a four-wheel drive, high-clearance vehicle to make the trek.

After a few miles, the road forks at a sign advising drivers that the next 3 miles are private property. Stay on the right fork at the sign, and buckle up. The road is rocky, bumpy, and bouncy all the way to the campground. These 8 miles could take you more than an hour to navigate, but they present you with the chance to see Pineview Reservoir and Cache Valley simultaneously. Now that's a view.

As your bones begin the last verse of the "Why are You Doing This to Me" chorus (that was Handel, right?), you'll come to a sign overlooking Willard Basin that talks about the rehabilitation of the canyon. Don't give up hope, you're almost there! A few more minutes to descend along the canyon's ridge, and you're there.

Willard Basin boasts a very unique landscape. The 1920s and 1930s saw uncontrolled flooding in the basin due to abuse of the land and fires that had destroyed much of the vegetation. After the flooding had caused two deaths and significant property damage, the local and federal governments stepped in to rehabilitate the land. They built fences, planted grass

RATINGS

Beauty: ✿ ✿ ✿ ✿ ✿
Privacy: ✿ ✿ ✿ ✿
Spaciousness: ✿ ✿ ✿ ✿
Quiet: ✿ ✿ ✿ ✿ ✿
Security: ✿ ✿ ✿ ✿ ✿
Cleanliness: ✿ ✿ ✿ ✿

and trees, and terraced the sides of the canyon to prevent further erosion and damages. Today the basin
calls to mind images of terraced rice paddies in Asia,
although it's a bit less dramatic than that.

Wildflowers, not wildfires, now blaze across the
canyon walls and floor, and everything in between. In
early August, bright reds, oranges, and whites carpet
most of Willard Basin, with the occasional clump of
purple- and pink-spiked accents. Where it's not painted
with color, Willard looks strikingly green—an interesting contrast to the rolling yellow and brown mountain-
sides found just to the east along the road in.

The campsites here are casual. If you've made it
this far on the torturous (but jaw-droppingly beautiful)
Willard Peak Scenic Byway, the Forest Service figures
you're probably not too concerned with comfort.
There are six sites, four of which have picnic tables.
Wherever possible they have been plopped down
among a stand of trees. Unfortunately, some of those
trees are ailing, so shade may become a rare commod-
ity over the course of the next few years.

Once you're staying in Willard Basin, you're
poised to capture some great memories on film. Take
the Willard Peak Scenic Byway to Inspiration Point,
found at the end of the road. It doesn't take a genius to
figure out how this spot got its name; there are phenomenal views of Willard Bay and the Great Salt Lake.
Somehow a wide-angle lens or panorama feature on
your camera won't seem to capture the awe you feel
standing there with such a unique perspective on the
West's most famous lake.

The Willard Basin Trailhead leaves near the
spring on the south side of the road at camp's
entrance. This trail will claw its way up to Willard
Peak, and eventually on to Ben Lomond Peak. Most
Ben Lomond peak baggers start from a different trailhead like North Ogden Canyon, but this route is actually shorter if you can stand the rocky ride in.

Even though the road keeps the big crowds out,
you'll probably still contend with OHVs at Willard
Basin. You might feel like Willard Basin is a remote
mountain retreat, but because it's still pretty close to

ADDRESS:	Wasatch-Cache National Forest Ogden Ranger District 507 25th Street, Suite 103 Ogden, UT 84401
OPERATED BY:	Wasatch-Cache National Forest
INFORMATION:	(801) 625-5306; www.publiclands .org
OPEN:	July–September
SITES:	6
EACH SITE HAS:	Fire ring
ASSIGNMENT:	First come, first served
REGISTRATION:	None
FACILITIES:	Spring water
PARKING:	Not assigned
FEE:	None
ELEVATION:	8,682 feet
RESTRICTIONS:	None

MAP

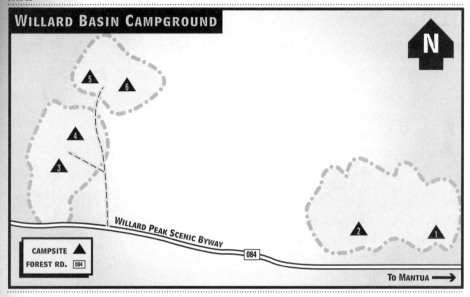

WILLARD BASIN CAMPGROUND

N

WILLARD PEAK SCENIC BYWAY

084

CAMPSITE ▲
FOREST RD. 084

To Mantua ⟶

GETTING THERE

From Mantua, go 8 miles south on the Willard Peak Scenic Byway.

some major population bases along the Wasatch Front, it does get a surprising amount of use.

Take extra care of the campground when you leave. You get the feeling that the rough access keeps the service project crews away, and it would be easy to see this location fall into disrepair. Tread lightly on the landscape to keep the wildflower shows as spectacular next year as they were the previous year.

I'm glad I've been to Willard Basin, and certainly feel like it's one of the great discoveries waiting to be had for all Utah outdoors enthusiasts. Someday I'll probably go back there to do some more hiking, snap some more photos, and spend a night or two in the unique canyon. It just won't be today. And tomorrow doesn't look too good, either. Maybe when my truck gets new shocks …

GPS COORDINATES

UTM Zone: 12
Easting: 418255
Northing: 4582738
Latitude: N 41.39202
Longitude: W 111.97779

5
LODGE CASEPGROUND

L ODGE **C**AMPGROUND HAS ABOUT ten big
brothers and sisters in Logan Canyon. It's this
status—as the runt of the litter—that makes it a
unique and charming little place for tenters to enjoy.

You'll find Lodge Campground off of US 89 just
east of Logan. US 89 deserves every bit of its status as
a National Scenic Byway. This winding highway makes
a dramatic cut through an awesome portion of the
Wasatch-Cache National Forest and demands the full
attention of every driver as it climbs and clings to towering canyon walls and carves through the cliffs high
above the Logan River below.

Lodge Campground is a refuge from all this
ruggedness—a safe haven found on a small detour up
the right fork of the Logan River. This is not to say that
Lodge isn't spectacular, just in its own way. While most
of Lodge's siblings give home to large amounts of
campers (Guinavah-Malibu has 40 individual sites), the
real charm of Lodge is in the fact that it has just ten.

Each of the sites here has just what you need—not
too much, not too little. A picnic table, fire ring, a
parking place, and a plot to plop your tent on. The
campground is laid out in a typical loop: sites 1
through 4 on the stem, 5 through 10 on the bend. Site
7 may have the edge on the others for privacy and spaciousness, but that's nitpicking, really. Each site here is
as good as the rest.

In contrast to the bigger campgrounds on the
main highway, you'll find more peace and quiet at
Lodge. Not only are you off the main road, but Lodge
remains somewhat undiscovered, or at least unfavored.
The only exception to peace and quiet would be traffic
coming to and from Camp Lomia, located only a few
hundred yards from the campground. It's a privately
owned camp used primarily for youth outings, so you
may catch a "drop-off" or "pick-up" day and have

> *US 89 deserves
> every bit of its status
> as a National Scenic
> Byway.*

RATINGS

Beauty: ✿ ✿ ✿ ✿
Privacy: ✿ ✿ ✿
Spaciousness: ✿ ✿ ✿
Quiet: ✿ ✿ ✿
Security: ✿ ✿ ✿ ✿
Cleanliness: ✿ ✿ ✿ ✿

KEY INFORMATION

ADDRESS: Wasatch-Cache
National Forest
Logan Ranger
District
1500 East US 89
Logan, UT 84321

OPERATED BY: Scenic Canyons

INFORMATION: (435) 755-3620;
www.fs.fed.us/r4/
wcnf/unit/logan

OPEN: June–October

SITES: 10

EACH SITE HAS: Picnic table, fire pit

ASSIGNMENT: First come, first
served

REGISTRATION: Self-register on-site

FACILITIES: Vault toilets,
drinking water

PARKING: At campsite only

FEE: $13 per night,
$6 extra vehicle

ELEVATION: 5,457 feet

RESTRICTIONS: *Pets:* Leashed
Other: 7-day stay
limit; 8 people per
site

plenty of company. Don't fret—it will soon be over and Lodge will return to its normal, peaceful self.

Shade is plentiful in and around the campground, which is good. At only 5,500 feet, it doesn't cool down as quickly as camps farther up the canyon. On the bright side, this means that the campground can open earlier and close later than many other Logan area camping spots.

As you drive up Logan Canyon, you may think to yourself that the Logan River looks like a great place to fling a fly. You're absolutely right. From the third dam on the river up to the Idaho state line, the Logan River is honored as a Blue Ribbon Fishery. This distinction comes with a price, however. Angler pressure is heavy, and special restrictions apply. Don't let that deter you. There's plenty of river for everyone, and even the kids can get in on the action a little lower at one of the impoundments closer to Logan City.

The right fork of the Logan River runs near the campground and is also a fun place to fish in its own right. Again, it's not as big or brassy as its big brother, the Logan River proper, but it is fishable.

If you take US 89 for 30 more miles away from Logan to see the Logan Canyon Scenic Byway to its end, you'll find yourself at Bear Lake. There are a few places to camp near the lake, but it's actually a great place to just spend the day even if you're based at Lodge. The lake is subject to vast fluctuations in water level, depending on the time of year and how wet previous winters have been, but it's usually pretty reliable as a place to hook into some Bear Lake cutthroat trout. This strain of the Bonneville cutthroat evolved in Bear Lake and now prospers in the alkaline waters of the lake.

Bear Lake is also famous for its raspberries, and in Garden City you'll see plenty of places to partake of the ripe red berries. If they're in season, bring some home for the neighbors and you'll be a hero for years. Don't miss the opportunity for a homemade raspberry shake, either. They're so tasty, most people have a hard time eating one slow enough to avoid a brain freeze. Be strong. Take your time. Savor the flavor; save a few brain cells. You may like them so much

MAP

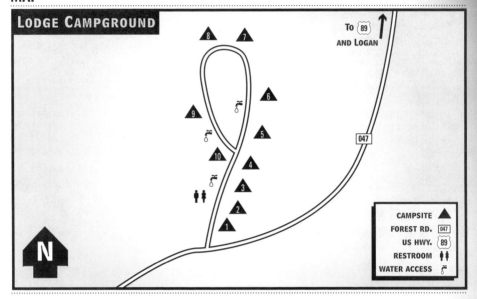

LODGE CAMPGROUND

To 89
AND LOGAN

047

8 7

6

9

5

10

4

3

2

1

N

CAMPSITE	▲
FOREST RD.	047
US HWY.	89
RESTROOM	♀♂
WATER ACCESS	

you'll have to get one on the way into town, and on the way out.

Logan residents who haven't yet discovered Lodge Campground will value its accessibility. Outsiders will welcome the straightforward layout and simple setup. Either way, the baby of the Logan Canyon campground family does the region proud.

GETTING THERE

From Logan, go 11 miles east up Logan Canyon (US 89), then turn right on Forest Service Road 47 following the signs to Camp Lomia. Continue 1.5 miles to the campground, just shy of Lomia.

GPS COORDINATES

UTM Zone: 12
Easting: 607075
Northing: 4523436
Latitude: N 40.85499
Longitude: W 109.72963

ONE WORD COMES TO MIND when describing High Creek Campground: rustic. There really isn't much of a campground here, at least not a formal one. Two distinct sites do exist, but it's the allure of High Creek Canyon itself that makes this area worthy of consideration. This is one of those rare places that only the locals know about, partly because they don't like talking about it, but mostly because they're the only ones within 50 miles of the campground.

Consider this: At High Creek, you're on the world-famous US 91 (huh?) between the thriving cosmopolitan city of Logan, Utah (what?) and Preston, Idaho (come again?). The campground is only 1.5 miles from the border of Idaho and about the same to bustling Richmond, population 1,849.

These are all good things. Very good things. This means that the rustic sites at High Creek and all the fun in High Creek Canyon aren't in any immediate danger of being overrun with people. Sure, you might find the occasional Scout troop on a Friday night, or a large group at the Lion's Grove (the local Lion's Club's day-use area), but if the campground's crowded there's plenty of opportunity for dispersed camping along the road.

So why come to High Creek? What the locals don't want you to know is that it's a fantastic place to begin your exploration of the Bear River Mountain Range. Zippy little High Creek makes its way down the mountain, beginning just below the upper reaches of the range. At the peril of my own life, I will divulge that there are indeed fish in this river, and they are, in fact, fun to catch.

High Creek also feeds the canyon with plenty of irrigation, so its shores are well shaded, even in the lowest reaches. Segments of the creek are lined with cliffs, others with brush. Fishing won't be easy here,

RATINGS

Beauty: ✿ ✿ ✿ ✿
Privacy: ✿ ✿ ✿
Spaciousness: ✿ ✿ ✿ ✿
Quiet: ✿ ✿ ✿ ✿
Security: ✿ ✿ ✿ ✿
Cleanliness: ✿ ✿ ✿ ✿

but for the persistent, the payoff can be surprisingly worthwhile.

High Creek flows right past the campground in some of its most accessible sections, so take advantage of the cool water. Even if only used for a few moments of contemplation, rivers are special things, and a campground with one so close shouldn't be taken for granted. Both sites enjoy the shade of the canyon walls and trees along the river. The small restroom is tidy and well kept. The campground is just about the only sign of civilization in the entire canyon.

The road past the campground continues to a point where a four-wheel drive is probably recommended. After you can drive no more, a steep trail continues up the mountain into the Mount Naomi Wilderness Area, and will eventually lead you right past High Creek Lake on the Naomi Peak Trail, delivering you down to Tony Grove Lake (see Campground #3). The whole trek is 10 miles (give or take), depending on how far up High Creek Canyon you trade in your tires for boot tread. It's a spectacular hike, rife with stream crossings, meadows, glorious views, and even bright wildflowers at the right time of year. Just don't be disheartened by the fact that your entire day of hiking into the forest leads you to a parking lot at Tony Grove Lake.

In the world of wildflower viewing, many people claim that the Bear River range is second to none. It isn't as accessible as some of the other contenders, so it probably doesn't get the same attention as places like the Albion Basin (see Campground #12), but the claim does deserve further investigation. You'll just have to come and judge for yourself. Shucks!

For an extended hike, take the fork of the trail that follows the north fork of the creek up Bear Canyon to the top of the mountain ridge and you'll find yourself in Idaho at the crossroads of several different canyons. You'll just have to explore them all to pick your favorite—White Canyon, Boss Canyon, Deep Creek Canyon. They're all gorgeous and inviting. Use caution in these canyons, however, as they're all steep and can become dangerous, especially if there's any snow or rain. Check the weather ahead of time, and consider bringing a good set of hiking poles for extra stability.

KEY INFORMATION

ADDRESS:	Wasatch-Cache National Forest Logan Ranger District 1500 East US 89 Logan, UT 84321
OPERATED BY:	Wasatch-Cache National Forest
INFORMATION:	(435) 755-3620; www.fs.fed.us/r4/ wcnf/unit/logan
OPEN:	May–September
SITES:	2
EACH SITE HAS:	Picnic table, fire pit
ASSIGNMENT:	First come, first served
REGISTRATION:	None
FACILITIES:	Vault toilets
PARKING:	At campsite or along road
FEE:	None
ELEVATION:	5,519 feet
RESTRICTIONS:	7-day stay limit

MAP

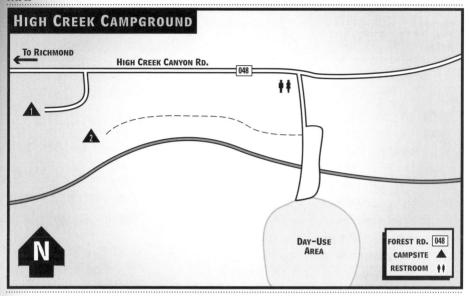

HIGH CREEK CAMPGROUND

To Richmond

High Creek Canyon Rd.

048

Day-Use Area

FOREST RD.	048
CAMPSITE	▲
RESTROOM	♀♂

N

GETTING THERE

From US 91 near Richmond, turn right onto 12000 North, which becomes 12200 North and eventually curves to 12400 North (High Creek Canyon Road/Forest Service Road 48). Go east a total of 5 miles to the campground.

Moose, elk, and deer wander the mountains in the Mount Naomi Wilderness Area, though they don't much make it down to the campground. Beavers are also abundant in many of the streams that amble down the local canyons.

You won't be swept off your feet by High Creek's high-class accommodations, but if you want a no-frills camping trip to an area where none of your friends have been, head up US 91 (huh?) towards Richmond (wait, where?) and into High Creek Canyon.

GPS COORDINATES

UTM Zone: 12
Easting: 439092
Northing: 4647421
Latitude: N 41.97643
Longitude: W 111.73517

7
MONTE CRISTO CAMPGROUND

FEW CAMPGROUNDS CAN RIVAL the "woodsy" feeling you get at Monte Cristo. Planted high in the Monte Cristo Mountain Range, the campground only opens for a few short months each summer, but year after year families keep coming back for the superb surroundings and fresh mountain air.

There are five loops at Monte Cristo and a total of 47 campsites. Only sites 26 and 27 can be reserved in advance, the previous being a group site holding a maximum of 80 people, the latter 100. The rest of the sites are only available on a first come, first served basis.

Ordinarily, a campground with 45 individual sites up for grabs gives you a decent shot at finding an open space. Because Monte Cristo is only open for three to four months each year, however, the camping season gets condensed and sites become scarce on a Friday afternoon. It's a wildly popular place to camp, for good reason. That just means you've got to get up there early to stake out your site.

Loop A or B will suit you just fine. Loop C is a good second choice. You'll probably want to avoid loops D and E if possible. They're closest to the big group sites and sit a little closer together than you'd hope. Each site has its own picnic table and fire ring, and only a few of the sites accommodate big RVs in pull-through sites. There's no river nearby to drown out the sounds of your neighbors, but if you're choosy about your campsite you'll be able to employ the "out of sight, out of mind" principle.

One of the reasons for Monte Cristo's popularity is its location—not only where it sits in the state, but where it sits on the mountain. Ogden and Weber County residents favor this place for its proximity to home. It's only an hour of so from Ogden City, but in terms of atmosphere, it's a world away. There are other fine campgrounds along the way, especially between

> *One of the best features at Monte Cristo is the symphony of scents in the air at any given time.*

RATINGS

Beauty: ☆ ☆ ☆ ☆
Privacy: ☆ ☆ ☆ ☆
Spaciousness: ☆ ☆ ☆ ☆
Quiet: ☆ ☆ ☆
Security: ☆ ☆ ☆
Cleanliness: ☆ ☆ ☆ ☆ ☆

KEY INFORMATION

ADDRESS:	Wasatch-Cache National Forest Ogden Ranger District 507 25th Street, Suite 103 Ogden, UT 84401
OPERATED BY:	Wasatch-Cache National Forest
INFORMATION:	(801) 625-5306; www.fs.fed.us/r4/ wcnf/unit/ogden
OPEN:	July–October
SITES:	47
EACH SITE HAS:	Picnic table, fire ring
ASSIGNMENT:	First come, first served; group sites reserved
REGISTRATION:	Self-register on-site; group sites online at www.reserveusa.com or (877) 444-6777
FACILITIES:	Vault toilets, drinking water, garbage service
PARKING:	At site only
FEE:	$12 per night, $5 extra vehicle
ELEVATION:	8,947 feet
RESTRICTIONS:	*Pets:* Leashed *Other:* 5-day stay limit

Pineview Reservoir and the junction with Causey Road. In fact, if UT 39 is still closed, there's a chance that one of these lower campgrounds will be open. Campers love that when UT 39 does finally open, there's a sheltered campground at 9,000 feet, located right off the highway, and that it's shaded by beautiful aspens and enormous evergreens.

This may sound odd, but one of the best features at Monte Cristo is the symphony of scents in the air at any given time. Whether it's after a rainstorm (somewhat common in these parts) or at dinnertime when families are cooking supper, the air here is always delicious. With the convenience of drinking water and garbage service, you can pack along the ingredients to the most elaborate camping fare and help contribute to the blend of splendid outdoors smells. Intoxicating!

Although there's no shortage of things to do, most people who stay at Monte Cristo really *stay* at Monte Cristo. The only deterrent you might have to lounging around your campsite would be the flies and mosquitoes. Some years are worse than others, but that just means the difference between bringing one or two cans of bug juice. You have been warned.

If you do have the willpower to break out of the Monte Cristo "aroma coma," drive to Birch Creek, about 12 miles away on UT 39 toward Woodruff. Two small reservoirs sit about a mile off the highway and are great places to dunk a worm. There's also a small campground with four walk-in sites operated by the Bureau of Land Management (BLM) if you just can't do the crowds at Monte Cristo.

Continue 2 more miles down UT 39 and turn off to Woodruff Creek Reservoir for similar recreational opportunities, minus the campground. This reservoir fluctuates greatly as the summer progresses, so expect muddy shores as fall approaches.

The Monte Cristo Range is full of back roads, byways, and little trails. As you drive along UT 39, duck into one of these turnoffs (once you've passed the private property segment) and see where it takes you. I took a trail just southwest of camp and found a cleared meadow that gave me incomparable views. I ended up snapping a remarkable photograph of the sunset, just

MAP

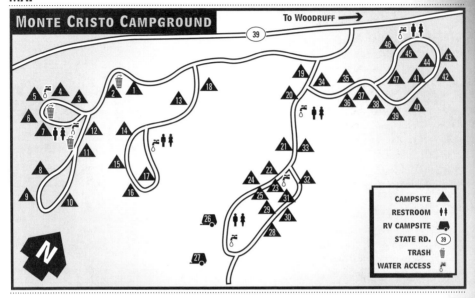

MONTE CRISTO CAMPGROUND

To Woodruff →

CAMPSITE ▲
RESTROOM
RV CAMPSITE
STATE RD. 39
TRASH
WATER ACCESS

as it dipped behind the mountains in the distance.

In the wintertime, this is a snowmobiling mecca. Ant Flat and Forest Service Road 054 (located just below the gate that closes UT 39 when the snow gets too deep) are buzzing with action. Monte Cristo Campground is closed, but the Forest Service does offer a wintertime cabin for snowmobilers, cross-country skiers, or snowshoers brave enough to make the trek. Accommodations are modest—propane heat, light, stove, and outdoor toilet (advertised by the Forest Service as "guaranteed to put hair on your chest") welcome the adventurous soul for just $40 a night. Call the ranger district directly for reservations.

GETTING THERE

From Woodruff, go 22 miles southwest on the Ogden River Scenic Byway (UT 39) to the campground.

GPS COORDINATES

UTM Zone: 12
Easting: 458437
Northing: 4590354
Latitude: N 41.46370
Longitude: W 111.49770

8
BOTTS
CAMPGROUND

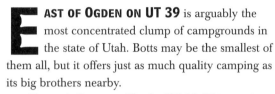

> *The south fork is one of the best places to launch an inner tube and float lazily downstream.*

EAST OF **O**GDEN ON **UT 39** is arguably the most concentrated clump of campgrounds in the state of Utah. Botts may be the smallest of them all, but it offers just as much quality camping as its big brothers nearby.

To reach Botts, you'll take UT 39. This two-lane road cuts through the narrow and winding Ogden Canyon area before opening up at Pineview Reservoir. As you pass by the south shores of Pineview, take note of the campgrounds you pass. These park and picnic grounds suit large RVs and boaters, but can become a little rowdy. Instead, keep going past Huntsville and leave the high-octane crowds behind. Soon you'll find yourself following the wide and rolling south fork of the Ogden River as you snake your way slowly up the Ogden River Scenic Byway. Here, open meadows and immense trees exist together in seamless harmony. Before you know it, you'll come to a small bend in the road and find Botts—the second campground on your right.

For all intents and purposes, Botts and Magpie could be considered as a dual entry. After all, the camp host for Botts stays in Magpie, and that's where you register and pay for the sites at both campgrounds. Botts, however, has just eight sites and a more laid-back atmosphere. That's not to say that it doesn't have its problems. Because the river and the road are so close together, Botts is sandwiched between the two and is consequently a little closer to the road than the ideal. The south fork does mute out some of the traffic noise, but not all. You'll also want to lock up your valuables and keep them out of sight to avoid being struck by a "smash and grab" criminal.

Each of the seven sites in the campground is immaculately kept. Site 8 must have been so well cared for that it was scrubbed away clean. I couldn't

RATINGS

Beauty: ✿ ✿ ✿ ✿ ✿
Privacy: ✿ ✿ ✿
Spaciousness: ✿ ✿ ✿
Quiet: ✿ ✿ ✿
Security: ✿ ✿
Cleanliness: ✿ ✿ ✿ ✿ ✿

find it on my visit. Perhaps you'll have better luck on yours. The main tables and campfire areas of each have recently been cast in cement and are as neat as can be. Next to the cement area is where you'll put your tent. There aren't actual tent pads, which is usually not a problem, but at Botts you'll probably have to get a little creative. Some sites have more obvious plots than others, though each is flat thanks to the topography of this river valley floor.

Botts is laid out like a curved needle, with restrooms and water in the middle of the small eye. Your best shot at staying away from your neighbor is in site 1, which is located immediately off the highway to the right. Site 2 is also set slightly apart from the rest and is a bit farther from the road. Site 7 is detached from the others and close to water and restroom facilities, but does back up pretty close to the highway.

Staying here puts anglers in the middle of some prime fishing area. Back down at Pineview, the reservoir flies in the face of the typical Utah trout fishery. While trout are still present, warm water species like bluegill, catfish, perch, and bass are more common targets. Pineview also boasts some of the biggest fish in the state with its healthy population of Tiger Musky, a sterile hybrid cross between a muskellunge and a northern pike. These fierce fighters are commonly reaching more than three feet long in Pineview.

If the buzzing boats and suburban feel of Pineview aren't your style, continue up the highway to Causey Reservoir. Causey has no developed boat ramp and holds nice rainbow, splake, and tiger trout, as well as a few kokanee salmon. Try near the inlets on either the Causey Estates or Boy Scout camp sides, but be cautious of current regulations. The inlets themselves have usually been closed for large portions of the year.

Truthfully, you don't have to go anywhere for fishing when you're staying at Botts. The south fork of the Ogden River holds some nice trout, especially the browns. You may have to fight for space on the river—although not with other fishermen. The south fork is one of the best places to launch an inner tube and float lazily downstream.

KEY INFORMATION

ADDRESS:	Wasatch-Cache National Forest Ogden Ranger District 507 25th Street, Suite 103 Ogden, UT 84401
OPERATED BY:	American Land and Leisure
INFORMATION:	www.fs.fed.us/r4/wcnf/unit/ogden
OPEN:	Mid-May–October (weather permitting)
SITES:	7
EACH SITE HAS:	Picnic table, fire ring, grill stand
ASSIGNMENT:	First come, first served; no reservations
REGISTRATION:	Self-registration at nearby Magpie Campground
FACILITIES:	Vault toilets, garbage service, drinking water
PARKING:	At campsite only
FEE:	$12 per night with 1 vehicle allowed, $5 each additional vehicle
ELEVATION:	5,250 feet
RESTRICTIONS:	*Pets:* Leashed *Fires:* In rings only

MAP

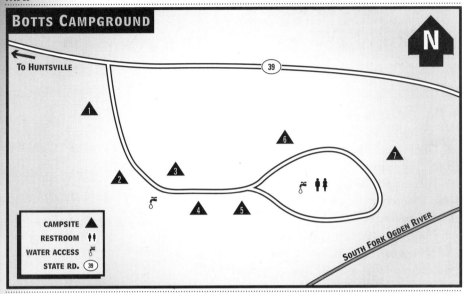

BOTTS CAMPGROUND

N

To Huntsville

39

1
6
7
3
2
4 5

CAMPSITE ▲
RESTROOM ♦♦
WATER ACCESS
STATE RD. 39

SOUTH FORK OGDEN RIVER

GETTING THERE

From Ogden, drive 12 miles east on UT 39 to Huntsville. The highway curves north, so turn right on 100 South in Huntsville to continue approximately 6 miles on UT 39 to Botts Campground on the right side of the road.

GPS COORDINATES

UTM Zone: 12
Easting: 444910
Northing: 4569748
Latitude: N 41.27729
Longitude: W 111.65780

Add an old inner tube to your list of camping essentials during the dog days of summer and you'll be rewarded with one of the finest ways to spend a hot afternoon. Let the cool and slow-moving waters carry you downstream until you pop out of your tube and walk up to do it all again. Massive cottonwoods around Botts provide shade for an afternoon snack before you head back upstream to give it another run. (How long do they tell you to wait before swimming after eating a meal?)

When you're all through at Botts, say good-bye and resolve to come back. There are enough campgrounds here that you could try a new one each time. Some are bigger. Some are farther from the road. But none have the unique charm of this little riverside campground.

9
BOUNTIFUL PEAK CAMPGROUND

A TWISTING ROAD TAKES YOU HIGHER and higher into Farmington Canyon on its way to a campground you'd never know was there unless you'd already heard of it. On its way, it moves from dusty and dry surroundings with barely a tree taller than you, to scattered oak in a few clusters, and finally to a patchwork quilt of quaking aspen and evergreens. This is Bountiful Peak Campground.

Designed as one giant loop, there are 29 campsites placed primarily among the aspen trees high in Farmington Canyon. The loop straddles a small hill, the first dozen or so sites on the upside, the remaining down below. You'll have to be careful when you select your site, because they're not all created equally. Try to avoid sites 6, 8, and 13. There are shadier and more private sites to be had. Numbers 5, 9, and 12, for example, are probably among the best this campground offers. Site 14 backs up nicely into a distinct bundle of aspens, and site 2 will require you to climb a few stairs to reach the table and fire area. The backside of the loop is where RVs have the best odds of parking, but they're not recommended at Bountiful Peak because Forest Service Road 007 is so narrow.

Precarious as it may be, you've got to love the road for what it offers in the view department. Early summer drivers get to see a verdant landscape coming to life, while autumn drivers are treated to a canvas of magnificent brushstrokes of foliage. And summer drivers can roll down the windows, rest their arm on the door, and feel the air becoming cooler and cooler as they make their way up into Wasatch-Cache National Forest.

Because 100 East in Farmington is such an unassuming little road, you really wouldn't expect to be able to follow it to a tree-packed campground. Not too many people stumble upon Bountiful Peak by

> *Autumn drivers are treated to a canvas of magnificent brushstrokes of foliage.*

RATINGS

Beauty: ✪ ✪ ✪ ✪ ✪
Privacy: ✪ ✪ ✪ ✪
Spaciousness: ✪ ✪ ✪ ✪
Quiet: ✪ ✪ ✪
Security: ✪ ✪ ✪ ✪
Cleanliness: ✪ ✪ ✪ ✪

KEY INFORMATION

ADDRESS: Wasatch-Cache National Forest Salt Lake Ranger District 6944 South 3000 East Cottonwood Heights, UT 84121

OPERATED BY: American Land and Leisure

INFORMATION: (801) 466-6411; www.fs.fed.us/r4/wcnf

OPEN: June–September

SITES: 29

EACH SITE HAS: Picnic table, fire ring

ASSIGNMENT: First come, first served

REGISTRATION: Self-register on-site

FACILITIES: Vault toilets, drinking water

PARKING: At site only

FEE: $10 per night, $5 extra vehicle

ELEVATION: 7,379 feet

RESTRICTIONS: *Pets:* Leashed Fires: In rings only *Other:* Closed 10 p.m.–6 a.m.

accident; in fact the only indication of anything interesting is a "Scenic Byway" sign along Main Street that's nearly completely faded white. Yet this campground has indeed been discovered. It has a full-time campground host—a rarity for a campground located so far away from pavement.

Despite its popularity and the lack of garbage service, the campground and adjacent areas seem to stay pretty and clean. Know ahead of time that everything you pack in, you've got to pack out. Plenty of people stay here every year and should be commended on their comprehension of that simple but sometimes elusive principle.

The summer months see plenty of campers traveling to Bountiful Peak, each for their own reason. Some are Davis County residents who want a quick respite from the sometimes scorching summer heat. Others are families who make it a tradition to camp here every year. Yet others still find Bountiful Peak as a more comfortable or at least budget-friendly alternative to hotels or campgrounds around Lagoon, the local thrill-ride amusement park. Whatever the reason, the campground offers a place for them all—or at least for the first 29 parties to arrive. It isn't the quietest campground in the state, but it's a lot calmer than any other campground for miles around.

Once you've made the drive to the campground, you may just want to hunker down and relax. That's fine, but if you've still got some driving left in you, go back to Skyline Drive and take it all the way south until it dumps you out into Bountiful City, more or less a few blocks north of the Bountiful LDS temple. You'll get a spectacular overlook of Davis County right below Bountiful Peak. You might also try the Francis Peak Road route (Forest Service Road 009) to summit Francis Peak. Things get a little dodgy toward the edge of the national forest boundary, so pay close attention to posted signs for the latest specific details.

Kids will appreciate the drive up to the campground. It's quite the setup for them to prepare for an outdoors adventure. And parents won't have to worry about water. There's plenty of H_2O on tap, but none in the immediate area that would pose a hazard to

MAP

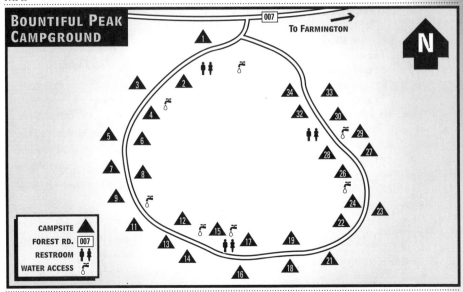

BOUNTIFUL PEAK CAMPGROUND

To Farmington

N

CAMPSITE
FOREST RD. 007
RESTROOM
WATER ACCESS

wandering little feet. Even on a day trip they'll be able to touch, smell, and see the outdoors. A $5 fee does apply for picnickers.

One group site exists at Bountiful Peak, and can be reserved online by visiting **www.reserveusa.com,** or by calling (877) 444-6777. It holds a maximum of 100 people and 20 vehicles. Call the Forest Service for the latest fee schedule.

GETTING THERE

In Farmington, take 100 East (which becomes Skyline Drive/FS 007) 9 miles east to the campground.

GPS COORDINATES

UTM Zone: 12
Easting: 432315
Northing: 4536922
Latitude: N 40.98066
Longitude: W 111.80456

10
REDMAN
CAMPGROUND

> *You could spend a week at Redman and do something different every day.*

THE DRIVE TO REDMAN CAMPGROUND is certainly striking: sheer rock faces full of daring technical climbers, a frothy mountain creek running along one side of the road and then the other, and more recreational areas than you could shake a hiking stick at. All of this on your way to the home base of high-mountain camping near Salt Lake City: Redman Campground.

This rather expansive campground is divided into two main sections: the upper section tucked into the channel between the highway and Big Cottonwood Creek, and the lower loop located on the other side of the river.

The upper section of Redman is where you'll find the camp host and, coincidentally, where you'll find most of the action. This campground is also a popular daytime and evening picnic spot, so cars pop in and out of the campground during most daylight hours. That could be a deal-killer, but the large acreage on which the campground is located helps dilute the perceived traffic congestion. Also, the upper section restrooms have recently been upgraded to modern flush toilets, whereas the lower loop still has a few vault toilets. The modern facilities of the upper area can be persuasive tools in helping you forget the crowds.

Still, if you like to get away from the buzz, cross the river and pick from campsites 23 through 49. This lovely bisected loop climbs the hillside and affords some of the more secluded camping in the canyon. If you don't have young children with you, take site 23 and the river will sing you to sleep each night as it passes through the edge of your site. To get as far away from civilization as possible, choose site 38, 43, or 44 on the back side of the loop where not too many vehicles or people pass.

RATINGS

Beauty: ✪ ✪ ✪ ✪ ✪
Privacy: ✪ ✪ ✪ ✪
Spaciousness: ✪ ✪ ✪ ✪ ✪
Quiet: ✪ ✪ ✪
Security: ✪ ✪ ✪
Cleanliness: ✪ ✪ ✪ ✪

Stretch out and relax at Redman, because there's plenty of land to call your own in practically every site. In a canyon dominated by pressure for development of private property, the Forest Service deserves kudos for allotting such a large chunk of land to campers. Don't get greedy with the spaciousness, though. Site limits on people and vehicles are strictly enforced.

As you enjoy the roominess of your site, look around and take in the scenery. The nearness of Big Cottonwood Creek means you get lush clumps of bright wildflowers and towering pines and aspens. Most sites will have a shady spot somewhere at all hours of the day.

In the mid-1800s, Big Cottonwood Canyon was explored by miners looking for gold, silver, and other precious metals. Today the real treasure of this back-yard canyon is the variety of recreational opportunities that it provides.

Redman sits between the two most popular trail-heads in the canyon. Just above the campground near Brighton Ski Resort is the boardwalk trail around Silver Lake. This easy stroll around the picturesque pond is accessible to everyone, even providing "piers" for handicapped-accessible fishing. Leave the boardwalk and climb the mountain trail behind Silver Lake to Twin Lakes, Lake Mary, and Lake Martha for more serene alpine scenery on a 5-mile round-trip hike. You can also access Lake Mary from a shorter, 1-mile trail that begins from a trailhead behind the Mt. Majestic Lodge in the Brighton Ski Resort area.

The other popular hike in Big Cottonwood Canyon begins back down UT 190 at the marked Mill B South Trailhead. Lakes Blanche, Florence, and Lillian will test your grit as you climb around 2,500 feet in less than 4 miles of the Twin Peaks Wilderness to these icy waters.

Doughnut Falls, a spectacular waterfall that cascades through a rock "doughnut," used to be a popular day-hike destination in the canyon, but was closed in 2004 by the owners of the property to "protect [their] private property rights." Although the majority of the trail is Forest Service land, do not trespass by going all the way to the waterfall.

KEY INFORMATION

ADDRESS:	Wasatch-Cache National Forest Salt Lake Ranger District 6944 South 3000 East Cottonwood Heights, UT 84121
OPERATED BY:	American Land and Leisure
INFORMATION:	www.fs.fed.us/r4/wcnf
OPEN:	Late June–September (depending on weather)
SITES:	43
EACH SITE HAS:	Picnic table, fire pit/oven
ASSIGNMENT:	Individual sites first come, first served; group sites reserved
REGISTRATION:	Self-registration on-site; group sites online at www.reserveusa.com or call (877) 444-6777
FACILITIES:	Vault toilets, drinking water, garbage service
PARKING:	At site, overflow at entrance
FEE:	$15 per night; $8 day use; $5 each additional vehicle
ELEVATION:	8,350 feet
RESTRICTIONS:	*Pets:* Prohibited *Other:* 8 people per site

MAP

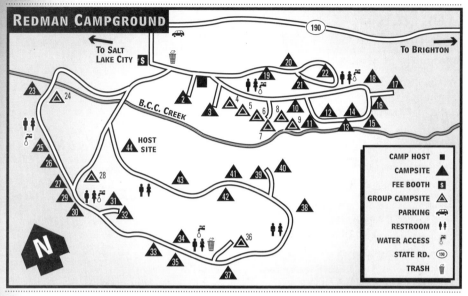

REDMAN CAMPGROUND

190

← To Salt Lake City S

To Brighton →

B.C.C. CREEK

HOST SITE

CAMP HOST	■
CAMPSITE	▲
FEE BOOTH	S
GROUP CAMPSITE	△
PARKING	🚗
RESTROOM	👫
WATER ACCESS	🚰
STATE RD.	190
TRASH	🗑

N

GETTING THERE

From Interstate 15, take the 7200 South exit east and go just more than 4 miles to the mouth of Big Cottonwood Canyon on 7200 South (which becomes Big Cottonwood Canyon Road/ UT 190). Continue east on the road 8 miles to the campground.

GPS COORDINATES

UTM Zone: 12
Easting: 450176
Northing: 4496239
Latitude: N 40.61547
Longitude: W 111.58901

You could spend a week at Redman and do something different every day. Besides hiking, this area of the Wasatch Mountains is a neat little place for fishing, mountain biking, photography, scenic drives, mountain climbing, and picnicking, and has even hosted a few kayakers, although the structure of the river is less than ideal for anyone but the hardcore paddlers. If camp cooking becomes tedious, stop by the Silver Fork Lodge for breakfast or brunch. Eat your omelet while overlooking the pines and aspens and you'll never want to eat indoors again.

Stop in at the Public Lands Information Office of the Wasatch-Cache National Forest for detailed recreation information. They're conveniently located inside of the REI store at 3285 South 3300 East in Salt Lake City, or available to answer questions by phone at (801) 466-6411. Take some of the free brochures and other information and you'll be able to plan a trip that maximizes all the activities in Big Cottonwood Canyon that will be at your fingertips in Redman Campground.

11
TANNER'S FLAT

AT TANNER'S FLAT CAMPGROUND in Little Cottonwood Canyon, convenience reigns supreme. Convenient location, convenient campsites, and convenient access to area attractions make this one of the easiest places to stay for your next camping trip.

Just 4 miles up the canyon, Tanner's Flat is probably the closest campground to most residents of the southern Salt Lake Valley. Drive to the campground and you'll notice that with each minute, you leave your cares behind and get carried away thinking about the trip ahead. Suburban lawns fade to grassy hillsides, stucco walls give way to sheer rock face, and soon you've gained nearly 3,000 feet in elevation. At 7,250 feet, Tanner's Flat is a welcome break from the hot summers of the city below, and lends itself to quick getaways designed to beat that heat. All this less than a half an hour from your driveway!

Tanner's Flat isn't just convenient for Salt Lake Valley residents. Most camping enthusiasts in Utah County can also make the drive in less than an hour and try something outside of the usual American Fork/Provo Canyon routine.

With camping made so easy, you'd expect this campground to be packed with people. Well, that's both true and untrue at the same time. It is true that the campground will fill up every weekend. There's a two-day minimum stay required over the weekends, so people come here to settle in, and once it's full, nothing will open up until Monday. But at the same time, thick clumps of aspen, oak, and pine form a barrier between the generously spaced campsites (with a few exceptions), so you'll be shielded from your many neighbors in this large campground. And although RVs are allowed, many RVers shy away from this campground because each site varies so dramatically in the size of RV it can accommodate.

> *Tanner's Flat is a welcome break from the hot summers of the city below.*

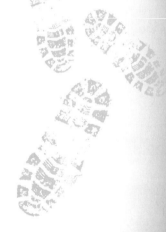

RATINGS

Beauty: ✿ ✿ ✿ ✿
Privacy: ✿ ✿ ✿ ✿
Spaciousness: ✿ ✿ ✿ ✿ ✿
Quiet: ✿ ✿ ✿
Security: ✿ ✿ ✿ ✿
Cleanliness: ✿ ✿ ✿ ✿

KEY INFORMATION

ADDRESS: Wasatch-Cache National Forest Salt Lake Ranger District 6944 South 3000 East Cottonwood Heights, UT 84121

OPERATED BY: American Land and Leisure

INFORMATION: www.fs.fed.us/r4/ wcnf/unit/slrd/ recreation

OPEN: Late June– September (depending on weather)

SITES: 38 plus 3 group sites

EACH SITE HAS: Picnic table, fire pit, grill stand

ASSIGNMENT: 13 first come, first served; the rest by reservation

REGISTRATION: Self-registration on-site; reserve online at www.reserve usa.com or call (877) 444-6777

FACILITIES: Flush toilets, drinking water, garbage service, amphitheater

PARKING: At campsite only

FEE: $16 per night, $5 each additional vehicle

ELEVATION: 7,250 feet

RESTRICTIONS: *Pets:* Prohibited *Fires:* In rings only *Other:* 8 people per site; gates locked 10 p.m.–6 a.m.; 7-day stay limit

The campsites here are easy to access. Upon entering the campground and passing the host's gatehouse, sites 1 through 19 are to the right down closer to the trout-stocked river, and 20 through 39 climb to the left. The road throughout the entire campground is paved, including the parking spurs for each campsite. The sites themselves are a bit on the small side, but you'll have just enough room to set up your tent and unpack the car. The only inconvenience is the placement of toilet facilities, as they're grouped near sites 7 and 9, and again near site 23. The only time you'll ever really notice, however, is when you first wake up in the morning after drinking too much soda the night before.

Sites nearest the entrance will naturally have more vehicle and foot traffic; sites 8 through 19 have pull-through loops instead of parking spurs, which will attract more RVs. Try staying at the far end of the upper section in sites 36 through 39 to avoid crowds. Reservation sites 3 through 6 will also keep you farther from the busy sections of the campground.

From Tanner's Flat you can jump off to one of several hikes in this popular canyon of the Wasatch Mountain Range. About a mile and a half farther up UT 210 you'll find the White Pine Trailhead. Shortly after this trail begins, it passes through an awesome visual reminder of the raw power of an avalanche. In the winter of 2004-2005, tons of tumbling snow came down the mountain across the White Pine Trail, knocking down everything in its path. Today the scar and the few lingering trees remain as a fascinating photo opportunity and chilling reminder.

If you've procrastinated deciding on a final destination for your hike, you'll have to make up your mind about a mile after the trailhead. The road forks at White Pine Fork Creek. Switch back left to go to White Pine Lake, or cross the creek right for Red Pine Lake. White Pine Lake is the longer hike at 9 miles roundtrip. Red Pine Lake is steeper, but only 6 miles roundtrip. Both are pleasant alpine lakes that are worth the 2,000-foot climb. If you want more lake for your buck, then go to Red Pine and keep climbing to Upper Red Pine Lake and the surrounding ponds. Both lakes are

MAP

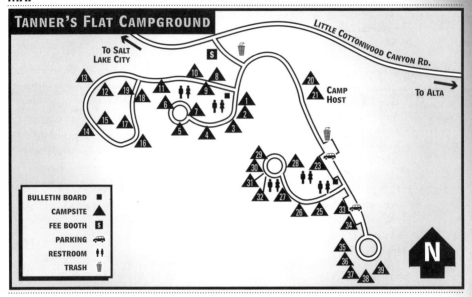

TANNER'S FLAT CAMPGROUND

LITTLE COTTONWOOD CANYON RD.

To Salt Lake City

To Alta

Camp Host

BULLETIN BOARD ■
CAMPSITE ▲
FEE BOOTH S
PARKING 🚗
RESTROOM ♀♂
TRASH 🗑

N

stocked with feisty cutthroat trout that can actually grow to a respectable size.

Farther up Little Cottonwood Canyon are more hiking opportunities: Hidden Peak, Maybird Gulch, Temple Quarry Nature Trail, and those near Albion Basin Campground (see Campground #12) to name a few. Check the Wasatch-Cache National Forest/Salt Lake Ranger District Web site, which has good information about each hike including length, altitude gain, difficulty, and description.

It's easy to get caught up in planning far-off and exotic camping adventures, but sometimes it's nice to slip away for a night or two without much thought. In those times, there's no better campground than Tanner's Flat.

GETTING THERE

From Sandy, take UT 209/9400 South (becoming 9800 South) east to the mouth of Little Cottonwood Canyon. Proceed east 4 miles up the canyon on UT 210 to the campground.

GPS COORDINATES

UTM Zone: 12
Easting: 440692
Northing: 4491476
Latitude: N 40.57194
Longitude: W 111.70068

12
ALBION BASIN CAMPGROUND

> *The Albion Basin is where Mother Nature shows off her artistic side.*

FOR A FEW SHORT MONTHS each summer, Albion Basin operates as one of the quirkiest little canyon campgrounds around. A perfect example of the stark contrast between commercial development and land preservation, this campground has a charm all its own.

At 9,400 feet, Albion Basin Campground is probably the last campground in Utah to open each summer. The Forest Service simply lists the opening date as July, although the campground may not open until mid- or late July after especially severe winters. Check with the Wasatch-Cache Recreation Information Center at (801) 466-6411 for the exact opening date.

Albion Basin is a typical single-loop campground, but that's the only thing typical about it. You could say that the campground is located in downtown ski country, as it's bordered by Alta Ski Resort. The resort's Albion Lift passes directly over the campground, and in winter the campsites are visited by skiers on their way down the mountain. In the summer, however, the ski lift sits quietly above the campsites as a powerful reminder to take advantage of each day of summer; winter is always waiting around the corner.

The campsites here are shielded well from each other, although I'd avoid sites 15 and 19. These two sites are set apart from other campers, but they're located next to private property with cabins well in view. The best sites are 22 through 24. Although closer together, they are removed from the considerable foot traffic generated by the nearby parking lot and trailhead that begins near sites 1 and 2.

That trailhead marks the beginning of the Cecret Lake trail. This 2-mile round-trip jaunt will take you up to around 10,000 feet, so be prepared to climb, especially in the last quarter of a mile. Don't be intimidated, though. It's common to see families with young

RATINGS

Beauty: ✪ ✪ ✪
Privacy: ✪ ✪ ✪ ✪
Spaciousness: ✪ ✪ ✪ ✪
Quiet: ✪ ✪ ✪
Security: ✪ ✪
Cleanliness: ✪ ✪ ✪ ✪

kids making the hike. There's nothing more embarrassing than being passed by a 6-year-old on the trail, so keep your legs moving and you'll soon be at picturesque Cecret Lake.

Despite its proximity to the town of Alta and the surrounding ski property, Albion Basin can take on a feeling of seclusion. Perhaps it's the immediate contrast of wild and domesticated land. Upon seeing the domesticated, you quickly identify yourself with the wild. It may be the small stream that wanders through the camp. Its slow-moving waters create just enough background noise to blot out the occasional sound of a passing car or group of hikers.

Or perhaps it's the brilliant and hypnotic wildflowers that carpet the surrounding hills each summer. Who has time to look at a ski lift when there are showy blooms of wild geranium, penstemon, Indian paintbrush and lupines in shades of purple, red, yellow, and white? The Albion Basin is where Mother Nature shows off her artistic side. There are hundreds of varieties of flowering plants in nearly every hue that delight visitors throughout July and August. Staying at the campground gives you a front-row seat.

If you're really excited about wildflowers, plan your camping trip around the Wasatch Wildflower Festival. This laid-back get-together of wildflower enthusiasts features several wildflower hikes with naturalists who know the area. Many also start with a tram ride up the mountain from a local ski resort, so the hike is all downhill. Live music and presentations help round out the event and make a great reason to get away. For more information, visit **www.wasatchwildflowerfestival.org.**

Albion Basin is also a popular place to start a mountain biking adventure. In the summer, the local ski resorts offer miles of mountain bike trails. Forest Service trails may or may not be open to mountain bikes, so check with the information center about your plans.

Don't be put off by the 3-mile dirt road into the campground. It's well maintained and family-car friendly. It will be a bit dusty, but the dust won't bother you much at your campsite. Along the road

KEY INFORMATION

ADDRESS:	Wasatch-Cache National Forest Salt Lake Ranger District 6944 South 3000 East Cottonwood Heights, UT 84121
OPERATED BY:	American Land and Leisure
INFORMATION:	www.fs.fed.us/ r4/wcnf
OPEN:	July–September (depending on weather)
SITES:	26
EACH SITE HAS:	Picnic table, fire pit
ASSIGNMENT:	First come, first served; group sites by reservation
REGISTRATION:	Self-registration on-site; reserve group sites online at www.reserveusa .com or call (877) 444-6777
FACILITIES:	Vault toilets, drinking water, garbage service
PARKING:	At campsite, overflow at trailhead
FEE:	$10 per night single; $20 per night double; $30 per night triple
ELEVATION:	9,400 feet
RESTRICTIONS:	*Pets:* Prohibited *Other:* 8 people per single site; gates locked 10 p.m.– 6 a.m.; 7-day stay limit

MAP

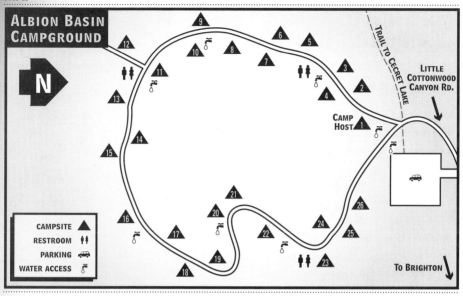

ALBION BASIN CAMPGROUND

N

CAMPSITE ▲
RESTROOM 🚻
PARKING 🚗
WATER ACCESS 🚰

TRAIL TO CECRET LAKE

LITTLE COTTONWOOD CANYON RD.

CAMP HOST 1

TO BRIGHTON

GETTING THERE

From Sandy, take UT 209 (9400 South, which becomes 9800 South) east to the mouth of Little Cottonwood Canyon. Proceed east nearly 11 miles up the canyon on UT 210, the road turning to gravel just past Alta Ski Resort for the last 3 miles.

GPS COORDINATES

UTM Zone: 12
Easting: 448094
Northing: 4492061
Latitude: N 40.57771
Longitude: W 111.61328

you'll notice a turnoff and parking area for the Catherine Pass trailhead. This trail takes you up through Catherine Pass for a magnificent view of Catherine Lake. Here you can press on toward the shores of Catherine Lake and farther to Lakes Mary and Martha, or you can continue climbing toward Sunset Peak. Numerous forks in the trail mean you can hike this area many times and always see something new. These forks also mean that investing in a good map will keep you from having an impromptu backcountry camping experience.

There are more remote and rugged campgrounds in Utah than Albion Basin, to be sure. But the convenience of sitting in your home in the Salt Lake Valley, and then setting up your tent high in Little Cottonwood Canyon just 45 minutes later just can't be ignored—neither can the spectacular wildflowers and backyard hiking experiences. Ski lifts and encroaching cabins? Well, they can be.

13
MILL HOLLOW
CAMPGROUND

THERE ARE NO SUPERLATIVES at Mill Hollow; it's not the highest, biggest, closest, or probably even most beautiful. But that doesn't mean it's a mediocre campground. In fact, it's the combination of great attributes that makes this little spot a must-see for Utah tenters.

Climbing the dirt road off UT 35 is a lesson in suspense. The road whips back and forth over graded (but washboard) dirt and never lets you see Mill Hollow Reservoir until you're within spitting distance. Then, you take an easy left over the dam and find yourself in the hearty forest campground on the shores of the light blue reservoir.

There are two simple loops: the elongated Loop A with sites 1 through 13, and the rounder, shorter Loop B with sites 14 through 28. Loop A is decidedly more spread out and has hiking access to the waterfront from a few of its sites. Specifically, sites 1 through 5 will get you closest, and site 5 is the most exclusive of the bunch. It can't be reserved, however. Only 4, 6, 8, 11, and 12 can be booked in advance in Loop A, sites 16 through 18, 20 and 21, and 26 in Loop B. For the others, plan a midweek trip or an early Friday arrival if you want to get a spot.

Some of the sites do accommodate RVs, but there's plenty that don't have a driveway and are better suited for tenters. The dense forest setting will help screen you from your neighbors. If you're concerned about getting a site that suits your tenting needs, numbers 18 through 20 are designated for tent use first.

In the farm- and ranching-favored west, where "whiskey is for drinking and water is for fighting," Mill Hollow Reservoir is something of an odd duck. It was created in 1962 and is maintained by the Department of Wildlife Resources and Uinta National Forest for recreational use. Where many other reservoirs capture

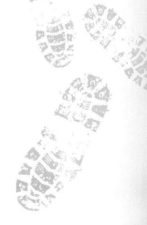

> *There are no superlatives at Mill Hollow.*

RATINGS

Beauty: ☆ ☆ ☆ ☆ ☆
Privacy: ☆ ☆ ☆
Spaciousness: ☆ ☆ ☆ ☆
Quiet: ☆ ☆ ☆ ☆
Security: ☆ ☆ ☆ ☆
Cleanliness: ☆ ☆ ☆ ☆

KEY INFORMATION

ADDRESS: Uinta National Forest Heber Ranger District 2460 South US 40 Heber City, UT 84032

OPERATED BY: Uinta National Forest

INFORMATION: (435) 654-0470; www.fs.fed.us/r4/uinta

OPEN: July–October

SITES: 28

EACH SITE HAS: Picnic table, fire pit, barbecue grill

ASSIGNMENT: First come, first served; reservations accepted

REGISTRATION: Self-register on-site; reserve online at www.reserveusa.com or call (877) 444-6777

FACILITIES: Vault toilets, drinking water

PARKING: At campsite only

FEE: $14 per night

ELEVATION: 8,887 feet

RESTRICTIONS: *Pets:* Leashed *Other:* 8 people per site

water in early spring runoff to release it slowly over the course of the summer for irrigation, water is never released from Mill Hollow for agriculture.

As a result, this is a tremendously popular family fishery. Angling pressure is heavy, but the hatchery truck makes frequent stops to deposit catchable-sized rainbow, brook, and albino rainbow trout. From the end of June through August, the lake is planted about once a week with one or more of those species, which average between 10 and 13 inches at planting time. While there is evidence that the reservoir has winter-killed in the past, most years it does not and any holdovers will start reaching the 14- and 15-inch plus range. That's no state record, but when little Tommy cranks in a 15-inch rainbow, he'll think it's the biggest fish that's ever flapped a gill.

Mill Hollow is also well suited to canoes and rafts. There is a crude boat launch, although no motors are allowed. If you just can't seem to find the fish from shore, or if the kids can't cast beyond the algae "gunk" that seems to form each season, bring your trusty vessel and paddle around to find an open space.

Explore the Mill Hollow trail that leaves from the campground to get better views of the surrounding canyon. After a few hundred yards the trail splits and lets you decide how tough you're feeling. Both directions will complete the loop, but the one on the left will take you through lodge pole pine and provides a more gradual ascent, while the fork to the right is much steeper and shorter. After you summit near a stand of aspens, the trail descends over steep terrain back down toward the campground, passing a small marshy area and joining a double-track road. While the trail is open to mountain bikes, they're not recommended because of the rough terrain.

If you continue on Forest Service Road 054 past Mill Hollow Reservoir, you'll quickly break out into an open mountain-top plateau crisscrossed with other backcountry roads. Continue straight on FS 054 until after it becomes Forest Service Road 094 and meets with Forest Service Road 050. You'll hook around on FS 050 and drop into the very beginnings of the west fork of the Duchesne River. Although it begins as just a

MAP

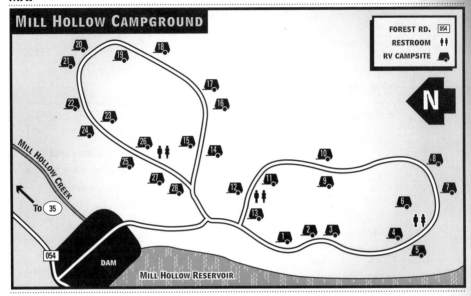

MILL HOLLOW CAMPGROUND

FOREST RD. 054
RESTROOM
RV CAMPSITE

N

Mill Hollow Creek

To 35

054

DAM

MILL HOLLOW RESERVOIR

trickle, you can follow the river as it picks up momentum from other small tributaries and local springs. By the time you've gone a couple of miles, it's turned into a bona fide waterway, teeming with little trout.

For as close as it is to the Wasatch Front, and how much it has to offer, it's a surprise that Mill Hollow isn't filled to capacity every night. Take advantage of this resource built for the very purpose of your recreation. You'll be glad you did.

GETTING THERE

From Woodland, go 11 miles southeast on UT 35 and turn right on FS 054. Drive south 3.5 miles to the campground.

GPS COORDINATES

UTM Zone: 12
Easting: 491211
Northing: 4482194
Latitude: N 40.49040
Longitude: W 111.10371

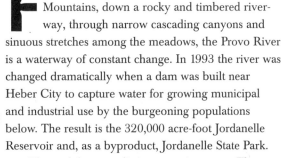

14
JORDANELLE STATE PARK–ROCK CLIFF CAMPGROUND

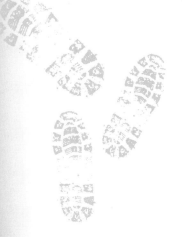

Leave your tent and you'll be angling at Utah's best fishing river in less than 60 seconds.

FROM ITS HEADWATERS HIGH in the Uinta Mountains, down a rocky and timbered riverway, through narrow cascading canyons and sinuous stretches among the meadows, the Provo River is a waterway of constant change. In 1993 the river was changed dramatically when a dam was built near Heber City to capture water for growing municipal and industrial use by the burgeoning populations below. The result is the 320,000 acre-foot Jordanelle Reservoir and, as a byproduct, Jordanelle State Park.

The park has two distinct camping areas. The larger and louder is the huge Hailstone complex, which hosts a marina, boat launch, restaurant, and day-use area complete with pavilions, beaches, and a playground. The colossal recreation complex on the western shore of the reservoir also holds ten distinct camping areas, with Keetley Point's 35 campsites as the only appointed for tent-only use.

Skip the madness and constant commotion that defines Hailstone and drive around to the Rock Cliff Campground on Jordanelle's southeastern shore. The Utah State Parks and Recreation division got it right here, creating a more tranquil alternative to Hailstone. All four campgrounds at Rock Cliff—Rock View, Upland Meadow, Aspen Grove, and Riverbend—are walk-in tent camping sites only, along the banks of the Provo River as it enters the reservoir. Park in one of the group parking lots and haul your gear over the boardwalks spanning the marshes below, and you can choose from 51 different sites tailored to a tenter's needs.

At 6,150 feet, this campground isn't exactly up in the alpine air, so the shade provided by the enormous riparian corridor cottonwoods is something to cherish. At Hailstone, they just don't have this luxury. The Rock View Campground (sites 1 through 7) was built to meet ADA standards and is closest to the parking

RATINGS

Beauty: ☆ ☆ ☆ ☆ ☆
Privacy: ☆ ☆ ☆
Spaciousness: ☆ ☆ ☆ ☆
Quiet: ☆ ☆ ☆ ☆
Security: ☆ ☆ ☆ ☆
Cleanliness: ☆ ☆ ☆ ☆

areas on the near side of the river. Reach Riverbend (sites 8 through 16), Aspen Grove (sites 17 through 36), and Upland Meadow (sites 37 through 51) by crossing the Provo River over a footbridge. Each site is clean and neat, spread out among the crisscrossing foot path.

Booking a site at Rock Cliff can be a confusing ordeal when done online. When visiting **www.reserve america.com,** you must enter "Rockcliff" as one word. "Rock Cliff" entered as two words (the correct way) doesn't find any matches, and "Jordanelle" will only pull up the sites at Hailstone. Sites 1 through 7, 17 through 23, and 45 through 51 are the only sites in Rock Cliff available by reservation, but your chances of getting a site by simply showing up are actually quite good, save for busy weekends and holidays.

Fishermen love the Provo River. It's the single-most fished river in the state, and with good reason. Here where it enters Jordanelle you'll find a good mix of rainbow and brown trout. Rock Cliff will make you feel like you're in a fishing camp of yesteryear—the kind where men wore flannel plaid shirts and had long bushy beards. Flannel-clad or not, leave your tent and you'll be angling at Utah's best fishing river in less than 60 seconds. Try throwing a small silver spinner upstream and zipping it back as fast as you can. Depending on the time of year, a bead-head prince nymph flung by a fly rod can catch the attention of cruising beasts.

The reservoir itself offers more family-friendly fishing. Standard baits seem to always produce a good rainbow trout or two, sometimes many more depending on the day. In addition, bass fishermen are now falling in love with Jordanelle for its recent ability to produce some beefy smallmouth. Pick up a copy of the latest fishing proclamation for complete rules on the area. Both the reservoir and the river have special regulations and are closely monitored.

If fishing isn't your game, you need not fear. Mosey on in to the nature center by the campground to learn more about the fragile wetland area around Rock Cliff and some of the creatures that call the area home. The nature center offers presentations in its theater nearly every day and campfire programs to help visitors deepen their appreciation for this special place.

KEY INFORMATION

ADDRESS: Jordanelle State Park
UT 319 #515 Box 4
Heber City, UT 84032

OPERATED BY: Utah State Parks and Recreation

INFORMATION: www.stateparks.utah.gov

OPEN: May 15–September 30

SITES: 51 walk-in sites

EACH SITE HAS: Picnic table, tent pad, fire pit

ASSIGNMENT: Group sites by reservation; individual sites first come, first served

REGISTRATION: Group sites call (800) 322-3770 or online at www.reserveamerica.com; individual sites self-register on-site

FACILITIES: Flush toilets, drinking water, fish-cleaning stations, nature center, small boat launch

PARKING: In group lots only

FEE: Individual sites $15–$18 per night; $75 minimum group fee plus $10.25 reservation fee; $7 additional vehicle fee

ELEVATION: 6,150 feet

RESTRICTIONS: *Pets:* Prohibited *Other:* 1 tent per site; gate locked 10 p.m.–6 a.m.

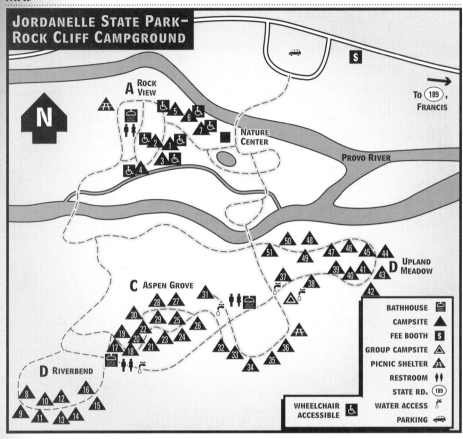

JORDANELLE STATE PARK—ROCK CLIFF CAMPGROUND

GETTING THERE

From Francis, drive 3.5 miles west on US 189 and take the marked turnoff to the campground.

GPS COORDINATES

UTM Zone: 12
Easting: 471363
Northing: 4494933
Latitude: N 40.60471
Longitude: W 111.33849

Birders flock to Rock Cliff (no pun intended) to see species like golden eagles, redtail hawks, and the nocturnal great horned owl that live in or visit in the region. The wetlands also host a bevy of big game including mule deer, elk, and moose. I visited on a weekday just after the campground had opened for the summer, and as I rounded a corner near the nature center, I found myself face to face with a big mama moose—only 15 feet away! After catching my breath, I got a great photo of the big beast and backed away slowly. I was later grateful for the tidy restrooms found at Rock Cliff.

With so much nature to see and experience in and around Rock Cliff, you'll hardly have a reason to leave. While it's sad to see that section of the wild Provo River now tamed, it has created new kinds of recreation and a terrific place to camp.

15
TIMPOONEKE CAMPGROUND

THEY SAY IF YOU LOOK at the profile along the peaks of Mount Timpanogas, you'll see the outline of a young Native American princess lying down in peaceful rest. Some people look at Timpanogas as the home of Utah's very own glacier. Still others see the rugged mountain as the home of one of Utah's most talked-about hikes. No matter what your angle, Mount Timpanogas is an awesome sight, and Timpooneke is the best seat in the house.

Timpooneke Campground is located less than 10 miles from Utah Valley, one of the fastest growing parts of the state of Utah. The increased population of Utah Valley has had a correlating effect on the tent population at Timpooneke. Once one of the hidden gems that no one ever knew about, Timpooneke has been discovered and reservations are almost a must now.

That's not to say that the campground isn't worth a visit or that you can't have privacy—you're just going to have to be smarter about how you do it. Because the campsites are spread out over a uniquely shaped layout, peace and quiet are still available to campers in the know. For starters, stay away from the loop located just before Timpooneke Road. These nine sites (6 through 14) are practically pinned to each other and would probably leave you wishing you'd stayed at another site. If you must, sites 6, 7, or 12 here are passable. If you're staying over the weekend, you'll be a bit frustrated in sites 4 and 5. They are accessed from the main parking lot of the Timpooneke Trailhead, which fills up early on Saturday mornings and has cars constantly coming and going all day. During the week, however, these double sites are actually quite nice. Your best bet for a quality camping experience enhanced by stunning views of the dramatic slopes of Timpanogas is on the back loop of the campground, in sites 15 through 30. The jewels here are sites 29 and

> *Mount Timpanogas is an awesome sight, and Timpooneke Campground is the best seat in the house.*

RATINGS

Beauty: ✪ ✪ ✪ ✪ ✪
Privacy: ✪ ✪ ✪
Spaciousness: ✪ ✪ ✪
Quiet: ✪ ✪ ✪
Security: ✪ ✪ ✪ ✪
Cleanliness: ✪ ✪ ✪ ✪

KEY INFORMATION

ADDRESS: Uinta National Forest Pleasant Grove Ranger District 390 North 100 East Pleasant Grove, UT 84062

OPERATED BY: American Land and Leisure

INFORMATION: www.fs.fed.us/r4/uinta

OPEN: June–September (depending on weather)

SITES: 30

EACH SITE HAS: Picnic table, fire ring

ASSIGNMENT: Some by reservation; others first come, first served

REGISTRATION: Reserve online at www.reserveusa.com or call (877) 444-6777; self-registration on-site

FACILITIES: Vault toilets, drinking water

PARKING: At campsite only

FEE: $11 per night, $22 doubles, $5 day use

ELEVATION: 7,300 feet

RESTRICTIONS: 14-day stay limit; gates locked 10 p.m.–6 a.m.

30, which don't have the views of the lower numbered sites, but are tucked back on their own little dirt driveway spur just above the main road.

You'll usually be greeted at each campsite with perky little alpine wildflowers that put on a dazzling display during July. Early in the year you may also be greeted by patches of snow. The camp is always scheduled to open on Memorial Day weekend, but the camp host recommends not making any definite plans until later in June, depending on the severity of the previous winter. Bugs greet every camper at every site. Flies are always around, and mosquitoes vary year to year from "thick" to "dense buzzing clouds."

Despite its newfound popularity and permanent pest population, Timpooneke just oozes charm. You'll wind along the Alpine Loop and see the canyon open up to stellar views of the valley below. In the fall, the road is full of Sunday drivers all week long, cruising for a chance to look at the brightly colored leaves. A small stream that runs through the upper loop of the campground looks like it comes straight from the snow-covered peaks above with the sole mission of gurgling for campground residents.

According to one version of the legend that named Mount Timpanogas, a young Native American princess named Uganogas fell in love with Timpanac, a stranger from another tribe, when he came to her father in search of food. Their love ended in tragedy when jealous braves from Uganogas's own tribe killed Timpanac by throwing him off of the mountain peak during a challenge the chief had created to award his daughter's hand in marriage. Devastated, the princess died of a broken heart and was buried on top of the mountain, her silhouette still discernible.

The same challenges issued to Uganogas's would-be suitors—running around a lake, hunting an animal, and climbing a mountain peak—are some of the main attractions of Mount Timpanogas today. American Fork Canyon has several lakes accessible to anglers. Try Tibble Fork Reservoir by heading 20 minutes back down the canyon and taking the fork on UT 144. This little reservoir is stocked with catchable rainbow trout that really come alive before dusk. Take the dirt road

MAP

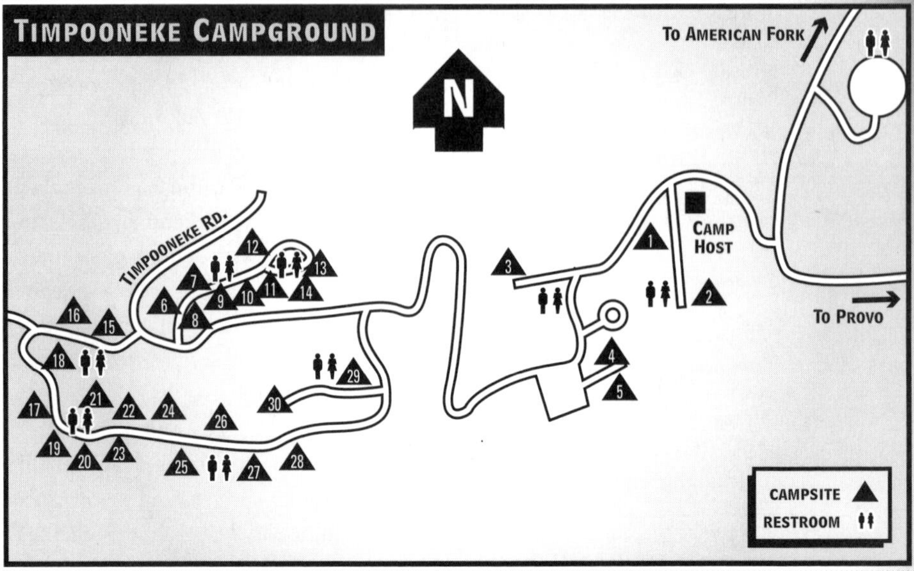

TIMPOONEKE CAMPGROUND
N
TO AMERICAN FORK
TIMPOONEKE RD.
CAMP HOST
TO PROVO
CAMPSITE
RESTROOM
1
2
3
4
5
6
7
8
9
10
11
12
13
14
15
16
17
18
19
20
21
22
23
24
25
26
27
28
29
30

from the Granite Flat Campground (located just above Tibble Fork Reservoir) to reach Silver Lake—a quieter, more challenging reservoir.

While you may not intend to hunt any animals, you'll at least see your fair share of them. Rocky Mountain goats, mule deer, moose, elk, and chipmunks are abundant in the 10,000-acre wilderness. You've also got a good chance of seeing mountain lions or black bears, so follow safe backcountry protocol.

If you've got a hankering to climb a tall mountain peak, Timp (as it's more commonly called) is *the* hike to do. There are two routes: Timpooneke trail, an 18-mile round-trip journey, and Aspen Grove trail, a 16-mile jaunt along much of the same trail. It has been suggested, however, the mileage marked overestimates the actual distance. Mileage notwithstanding, you'll gain nearly 5,000 feet in elevation and it will take you the better part of the day. Be prepared for a long hike and be aware of rapidly changing weather that can drive you off the mountain. If you're not in for the long haul, try Timpanogas Cave National Monument, an easy foot path to a large cavern near the mouth of American Fork Canyon.

GETTING THERE

Drive south on Interstate 15 from Salt Lake City and take the Highland/Alpine/UT 92 exit for 5.5 miles. Continue on UT 92 (the Alpine Loop) for 9 miles up American Fork Canyon.

GPS COORDINATES

UTM Zone: 12
Easting: 446018
Northing: 4476077
Latitude: N 40.4336
Longitude: W 111.6364

> *Stay at Hope and you can hop back to camp to change clothes, grab a bite to eat, swap your gear, and head back out to play.*

T'S HARD TO KEEP FROM GIGGLING when you make the turn off of US 189 toward Squaw Peak. Almost everyone in Utah County knows that Squaw Peak is where the local young couples go to spend "quality time" together. What no one seems to know, though, is that the road to Utah County's veritable "Lover's Lane" also takes you to one of Utah's best-kept camping secrets: Hope Campground.

Hope Campground is just minutes away from the immediate Provo/Orem area, so you'd expect it to be jammed with people looking for a quick weekend getaway. It's the only overnight campground located in the immediate Provo Canyon area, after all. How delightful, then, to discover you've got a good chance at finding a vacancy among the 24 sites here, even on a weekend. Also, the road forks below the campground, sending sweethearts one way and serious campers the other.

With a name like Hope, you may be tempted to run up the canyon and look for an empty site. Although it's likely your hopes become reality, reservations are accepted on all but two of the sites here (sites 1 and 2), so you should still probably try to book ahead of time. Family reunions or large group activities can fill this camp quickly; better to be safe than sorry.

After leaving the pavement above the campground, you'll descend on a dirt road to find the sites. Hope is a long oval loop cut down the middle with another straight road. There are campsites along the outer loop on both sides of the road, as well as both sides of the bisecting road. The sites here sit under a shady mixture of oak and a few maple trees. At 6,600 feet you're not quite in pine tree territory, so you definitely don't get a high mountain feel. That's most evident during sizzling daytime hours when the temperature can still be a hair on the hot side.

RATINGS

Beauty: ✪ ✪ ✪ ✪
Privacy: ✪ ✪ ✪
Spaciousness: ✪ ✪ ✪
Quiet: ✪ ✪ ✪ ✪
Security: ✪ ✪ ✪ ✪
Cleanliness: ✪ ✪ ✪ ✪

You won't have extreme privacy at Hope, but you won't feel like your personal space is constantly being invaded either. Site 3 is above the road to the left as you first enter and would allow you to hide your tent away quite nicely. Park at site 8 and you'll climb a few stairs and disappear behind some of the low-growing vegetation. Conversely, site 5 is right on the road and would make you feel like you could be run over at any minute while sitting in your tent. You'll also find good access to water everywhere around the campground, except in the bend around sites 10 and 11. Although there is a small creek that runs through the bottom of Pole Canyon to the east, you can only access it by foot on the steep shores. Having water available right in camp is a real blessing.

Provo Canyon is a popular place for many different reasons. Families flock to the area for its many parks and places to picnic and play. Teens and college kids come to float the Provo River in an inner tube and, inevitably, have a water fight. Anglers are in love with the Provo River for the big browns and rainbows it's been known to churn out. It's Utah's most popular stretch of river, deserving every bit of its Blue Ribbon status. Paddlers get in on the action for the long, smooth beginner rides available in several stretches in the canyon. The Provo River Parkway Trail, a paved walkway along the shores, draws in-line skaters, bikers, and exercise enthusiasts looking for change of pace. Stay at Hope and you can hop back to camp to change clothes, grab a bite to eat, swap your gear, and head back out to play. Just be mindful of private property lines along the canyon—there are quite a few. When in doubt, stick to the specially marked public access areas.

Be sure to visit Bridal Veil Falls, just up the canyon from Squaw Peak road along US 189. This spectacular 607-foot waterfall cascades over layers of rock on its way to a small and enchanting pool along the canyon floor. Drive right to the pool area and kink your neck trying to follow a single drop as it twists, turns, crashes, and tumbles its way down. You'll also see the remains of a tramway that once held the distinctive honor of being the world's steepest tram—now out of operation due to avalanche damage in 1997.

KEY INFORMATION

ADDRESS:	Pleasant Grove Ranger District 390 North 100 East Pleasant Grove, UT 84062
OPERATED BY:	American Land and Leisure
INFORMATION:	www.fs.fed.us/r4/uinta
OPEN:	Late May–October (depending on weather)
SITES:	24
EACH SITE HAS:	Picnic table, fire ring, barbecue stand
ASSIGNMENT:	Some by reservation; others first come, first served
REGISTRATION:	Reserve online at www.reserveusa.com or call (877) 444-6777; self-registration on-site
FACILITIES:	Vault toilets, drinking water
PARKING:	At campsite only
FEE:	$11 per night; $22 doubles; $5 day use
ELEVATION:	6,660 feet
RESTRICTIONS:	Gates locked 10 p.m.–6 a.m.

MAP

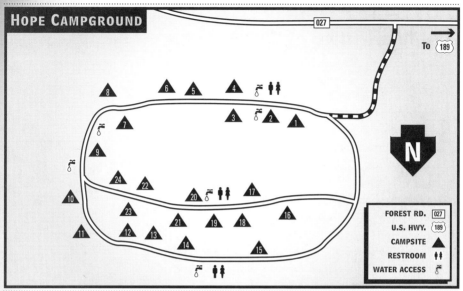

HOPE CAMPGROUND

GETTING THERE

From Orem, take US 189 2 miles up Provo Canyon. Turn south on Squaw Peak Road and go 5 miles to the campground.

If you were to ask the typical Squaw Peak visitor what's at the end of Squaw Peak Road, more than one would probably say "hope" of some kind. Little do they (and most others) know that's the name of an inviting little campground just minutes from the noise of Utah County.

GPS COORDINATES

UTM Zone: 12
Easting: 447374
Northing: 4461759
Latitude: N 40.3047
Longitude: W 111.6193

17
BUTTERFLY LAKE CAMPGROUND

DRIVE THROUGH THE Uinta Mountains along Mirror Lake Highway (UT 150) and you may be tempted to stop at one of the many campsites before reaching Mirror Lake; there are 12. Do yourself a favor and continue to lucky number 13— Butterfly Lake Campground. It's worth the extra few minutes on one of Utah's most breathtaking scenic byways.

Nestled against Butterfly Lake and tucked into towering pines, this road and single-loop campground has 20 sites, water, and vault restroom facilities. Arrive early and have your pick of meadow sites (14 through 16), lakefront sites (17 through 19), or more secluded sites (1 through 3). The remaining sites are located around the loop in a typical wooded setting, although the healthy amount of space allotted to each is anything but typical for the Mirror Lake Highway area. Here you can spread out a bit and exhale.

From your campsite at Butterfly Lake your biggest problem may be choosing which adventures to take. The Uinta Mountains are the only major mountain range in the contiguous United States that run east to west. With hundreds of rivers and small streams, and more than a thousand lakes dotting the map, these mountains hold millions of adventures to be had by the willing camper.

If hiking is on your agenda, then this campground makes an excellent point for launching off. For an easy, family-friendly hike, make your way to the Ruth Lake Trailhead about a mile farther down UT 150. The 1.5-mile round-trip trail is well marked and gains only 200 feet in elevation. Fishing and exploring are popular pastimes at Ruth Lake.

If you want more of a challenge than Ruth Lake has to offer, make your way 8.5 miles back on UT 150 to the Crystal Lake Trailhead, located just beyond the

> *These mountains hold millions of adventures to be had by the willing camper.*

RATINGS

Beauty: ✩ ✩ ✩ ✩ ✩
Privacy: ✩ ✩ ✩ ✩
Spaciousness: ✩ ✩ ✩ ✩ ✩
Quiet: ✩ ✩ ✩
Security: ✩ ✩ ✩ ✩
Cleanliness: ✩ ✩ ✩ ✩

KEY INFORMATION

ADDRESS: Butterfly Lake Campground Wasatch-Cache National Forest 50 East Center Street Kamas, UT 84036

OPERATED BY: American Land and Leisure

INFORMATION: www.fs.fed.us/r4/ wcnf/unit/kamas

OPEN: Memorial Day–Labor Day (depending on weather)

SITES: 20

EACH SITE HAS: Picnic table, fire ring

ASSIGNMENT: First come, first served

REGISTRATION: Self-register on-site

FACILITIES: Vault toilets, drinking water

PARKING: At campsite only

FEE: $12 per night, $5 day use; recreation pass required: $3 per day, $6 per week, $25 per year

ELEVATION: 10,290 feet

RESTRICTIONS: *Fires:* In rings only *Other:* 14-day stay limit

tightly packed RVs common at the Washington Lake Campground. Once at the Crystal Lake Trailhead, park and pick your poison. This trailhead hosts three separate hikes. For scenery, go with the hike to Island Lake along the Smith-Morehouse trail. It's 3.5 miles each way and passes several lakes, meadows, and mountain views.

For even more impressive views of lakes dotting the entire mountain landscape, start on the trail to Crystal Lake and take the marked fork past Cliff, Petit, Linear, Watson, and Clyde Lakes. Another ten lakes are within striking distance from Clyde.

Marjorie and Weir Lakes both hold arctic grayling. Though small, these feisty fish are a treat for the angler who has never caught one. Follow the Smith-Morehouse trail over the Mt. Watson pass and then fork left at the trail marker.

For a more relaxing activity, try strolling around the southern tip of Mirror Lake on the boardwalk, or picnicking back on Bald Mountain Pass. You're sure to have neighbors at both, but the views are worth it. Ten miles back from Butterfly Lake is Provo River Falls. Park in the designated turnoff and see the water cascade over staircases of slate. Bring a camera for sure!

Don't feel like you have to leave Butterfly Lake to take advantage of what the Uintas have to offer. Although fished frequently, Butterfly still holds willing albino, rainbow, and brook trout. It's stocked regularly and the fish can be coaxed onto your line with small lures or classic worm rigs.

It's been said that being a weatherman in the Uintas is the easiest job in Utah; their line: "It will be gorgeous … until it's not." The weather can change unexpectedly, and brief afternoon rainstorms are the rule more than the exception. Come prepared and you'll welcome a few raindrops. Come *un*prepared and you'll find out just how many ways there are to say "damp." At an elevation of more than 10,000 feet, winter snow lasts until June or July, so call ahead to see if the highway and campgrounds are cleared and open.

Butterfly Lake Campground is only two hours from Salt Lake City, so even here crowds can be an issue. Holidays, especially the Fourth of July and Labor Day, are extremely busy along the Mirror Lake Highway.

MAP

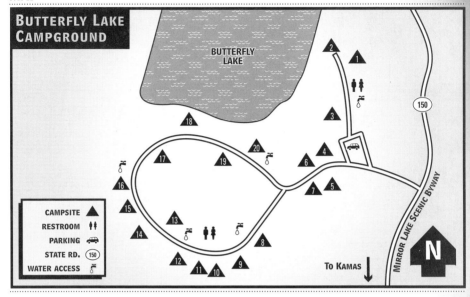

BUTTERFLY LAKE CAMPGROUND

BUTTERFLY LAKE

150

18
20
17
19
16
15
13
14
12
11
10
9
8
5
7
6
4
3
1
2

CAMPSITE ▲
RESTROOM
PARKING
STATE RD. 150
WATER ACCESS

To KAMAS

MIRROR LAKE SCENIC BYWAY

N

Leave home early if you're planning to camp during one of those weekends. During other weekends and especially weekdays, however, you'll find Butterfly Lake Campground to be the perfect hideaway in the spectacular Uinta Mountains.

On your way home, stop at "Dick's Café," located just down from the high school as you're headed back into Kamas on the edge of town. Get a double bacon cheeseburger, fries, and chocolate banana shake for the perfect ending to your trip.

GETTING THERE

Take Interstate 80 to Exit 156 (UT 32 Wanship/Kamas). Go south on UT 32 for 16 miles to the town of Kamas. Turn Left at Center Street in Kamas on UT 150 (Mirror Lake Scenic Byway) and continue 34 miles to Butterfly Lake Campground.

GPS COORDINATES

UTM Zone: 12
Easting: 511199
Northing: 4507757
Latitude: N 40.72066
Longitude: W 110.86740

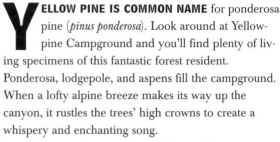

> *This campground is functional and friendly to campers of all levels of ability.*

YELLOW PINE IS COMMON NAME for ponderosa pine (*pinus ponderosa*). Look around at Yellowpine Campground and you'll find plenty of living specimens of this fantastic forest resident. Ponderosa, lodgepole, and aspens fill the campground. When a lofty alpine breeze makes its way up the canyon, it rustles the trees' high crowns to create a whispery and enchanting song.

Tucked just below Upper Stillwater Reservoir in the midst of all these trees, Yellowpine Campground has one attribute that so few other campgrounds can boast: accessibility. I'm not just talking about the paved road that takes you there (although that sinuous stretch of road that rambles along Rock Creek is undoubtedly accessible to any driver), I'm talking about the accessibility of the campground facilities to campers with disabilities.

The Forest Service has put forth an obvious effort to ensure that this campground is functional and friendly to campers of all levels of ability. The entire campground loop is paved, as are the walkways to and from each paved picnic table and fire ring area. There's also a paved nature trail and wooden fishing dock near the campground that open up a world of possibilities not always available at other campgrounds.

Before you go thinking the entire place looks more like a paved supermarket parking lot than a campground, take into account the efforts of Mother Nature to provide a real outdoors experience. The massive trees make such little pavement look inconsequential, so you really don't much notice the asphalt beneath you.

One of the best ways to identify ponderosa and lodgepole pines is by their tall, straight trunks—lodgepoles more so than ponderosas. They typically have fewer branches near the ground, which means

RATINGS

Beauty: ✿ ✿ ✿ ✿
Privacy: ✿ ✿ ✿
Spaciousness: ✿ ✿ ✿ ✿ ✿
Quiet: ✿ ✿ ✿ ✿ ✿
Security: ✿ ✿ ✿ ✿ ✿
Cleanliness: ✿ ✿ ✿ ✿ ✿

that campsites here aren't as private as they might be in the presence of say, firs or cedars. That's OK. You'll find *enough* privacy to be comfortable.

Both species of trees have been an important part of Utah's history. Lodgepoles, found primarily here in the Uintas, were used extensively in the state's early years for railroad ties and as poles for fences. They're still used as a pine lumber for construction. Ponderosas are a highly utilized timber for mill products today, just as they were in the days when Utah was being settled. Before that time, the Nez Pierce and Crow used the pitch for glue, and the Cheyenne applied it to the inside of their flutes to improve the sound.

The first 17 sites on the loop can be reserved through the National Recreation Reservation Service. The remaining 12 sites are first come, first served. You'll probably want to book plenty in advance, although I was surprised on my visit to see only a handful of spots were taken. Then again, that's the beauty of showing up on a Thursday afternoon.

Rock Creek itself provides pretty good fishing opportunities—rainbows and browns mostly. There are even a few good pools on the south fork of Rock Creek as it enters Rock Creek proper, but only for a mile or so. The upper reaches of the south fork are gorgeous but devoid of fish—probably due to natural barriers in the river created by avalanches and a steep riverbed.

Don't let the lack of fish discourage you from taking the dirt road up the south fork. The river is gorgeous up that high and a pleasure just to view. From just below the Upper Stillwater Campground (currently closed due to hazardous trees), take Forest Service Road 134 to its fork with Forest Service Road 143. From there, FS 143 follows the south fork and eventually plants you at a vague trail to Arta and Survey Lakes. These are both planted with little trout but often winter-kill in severe winters. The hike is short but steep to Arta—the same from Arta to Survey. Again though, even fishless there's plenty of reason to come here.

FS 134 will actually take you over the mountain and back down again before it reconnects with UT 35

KEY INFORMATION

ADDRESS:	Ashley National Forest Duchesne Ranger District 85 West Main Duchesne, UT 84021
OPERATED BY:	Ashley National Forest
INFORMATION:	(435) 738-2482; www.fs.fed.us/r4/ashley
OPEN:	May–September
SITES:	29
EACH SITE HAS:	Picnic table, fire ring
ASSIGNMENT:	First come, first served; reservations accepted
REGISTRATION:	Self-register on-site; reserve online at www.reserveusa.com or call (877) 444-6777
FACILITIES:	Modern toilets, drinking water, garbage service
PARKING:	At campsite only
FEE:	$10 per night
ELEVATION:	7,601 feet
RESTRICTIONS:	*Pets:* Leashed

MAP

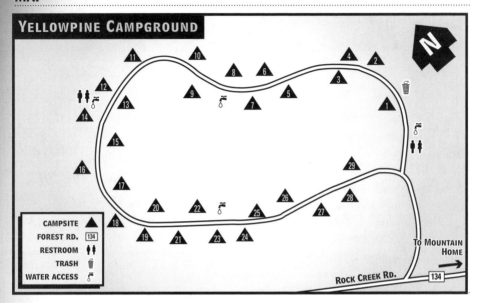

YELLOWPINE CAMPGROUND

CAMPSITE ▲
FOREST RD. 134
RESTROOM
TRASH
WATER ACCESS

To MOUNTAIN HOME →

ROCK CREEK RD. 134

GETTING THERE

From Mountain Home, take Rock Creek Road (FS 134) 20 miles northwest to the campground.

near Hannah. If you're looking for a different way home or a scenic drive, this is an excellent choice. There's even a brief, Bryce Canyon-esque feel to the cliffs on the north side of the mountain ridge where a jagged outcropping of spires clings to the solid cliff wall behind it. It's a magnificent route, but it does require a high-clearance vehicle.

You don't have to be a dendrologist (a tree geek) to enjoy Yellowpine. In fact, that's what makes it so valuable—it can be enjoyed by so many people for so many different reasons.

GPS COORDINATES

UTM Zone: 12
Easting: 530685
Northing: 4487259
Latitude: N 40.53551
Longitude: W 110.63768

NOT TOO MANY PEOPLE could tell you where Hobble Creek is. Those who do would probably say, "Ya. I golfed there." The next time you go up Hobble Creek Canyon, take the golf clubs out of your car and make room for a tent and sleeping bag, because Balsam Campground is a superb place to camp.

Hobble Creek runs through a small canyon east of Springville—not the biggest creek or the biggest canyon. The campground is often passed over for consideration by campers who opt for the highest mountain, deepest lake, or lowest valley. Those campers can have their superlatives, because what Hobble Creek Canyon does offer is a tranquil and serene setting for campers who love their solitude.

The campsites at Balsam are spread out along the banks of Hobble Creek—some of which you will only be able to access by foot bridge. That means that tent camping reigns supreme here. Enter the camp from Canyon Drive and you'll immediately see the group camping section to your right. A large parking lot and vault toilets sit on a small plateau above the river. Keep on the main road and pass the host to find the individual campsites. After passing site 1, you'll cross Hobble Creek on a small bridge and come to a small parking area. Through the woods behind the parking area is site 3, one of the most private in this campground. If the triple site (site 6) is unoccupied, site 3 will be quiet and put you close to the amenities. However, groups at site 6 tend to expand the limits of their campsite until it bulges to the borders of site 3. Sites 13 through 16 are your safest bet for isolation. Park at the round parking lot at the end of the main road and walk in to these tent-only sites. They're removed from the river, but it's worth the sacrifice to be tucked into the oak and maples in this section of the campground.

> *What Hobble Creek Canyon does offer is a tranquil and serene setting for campers who love their solitude.*

RATINGS

Beauty: ✿ ✿ ✿ ✿
Privacy: ✿ ✿ ✿ ✿
Spaciousness: ✿ ✿ ✿
Quiet: ✿ ✿ ✿
Security: ✿ ✿ ✿ ✿
Cleanliness: ✿ ✿ ✿ ✿

You'll notice that there are two footbridges along-side the camp road. Both lead to campsites across the river, but access to the first set (sites 17 through 24) is actually alongside the main canyon road in a large parking area. These sites are removed from the rest of camp, but unfortunately they're a little too close together and probably too close to the road for real comfort. The second set, sites 8 and 9, are a little more relaxed.

Pay attention to the road when you're finding your way to Balsam Campground. After turning up 400 South, you'll come to a three-way stop sign. Make sure you turn to the right toward the golf course. After passing the golf course, turn right or you'll shoot by the canyon.

Hobble Creek has quietly become a favorite little spot for fly-fishermen looking to be driven mad. It's a small creek with a lot of underbrush and wary little trout. If you plan on fishing here, bring plenty of tippet and extra flies; you'll probably end up decorating a few trees with hand-tied dry fly ornaments. Sneak up on a fish, give the perfect presentation, watch him slurp your offering, and you'll definitely forget the frus-tration of losing a little gear.

You won't find many obvious hiking opportunities in the canyon, but the dedicated hiker will still find a few trails to explore. The main hike in the canyon begins at the trailhead where Wardsworth Creek enters Hobble Creek, just a minute up the road from Balsam. Take the trail for 3 miles along Wardsworth Creek to a small stock pond. Here you have the option of either turning around, joining the Dry Creek Canyon trail to make a loop, or continuing on to Halls Fork Road. If you take the trail to its end, you'll actually end up on the Great Western Trail near Twin Peaks and then Daniel's Summit in Wasatch County.

If you've got room in your car for both camping gear and golf clubs, throw them both in. Hobble Creek is a beautiful canyon golf course that runs parallel to the river and is flanked by tall trees on both sides, with Gambel Oak stands throughout.

After delivering you to Balsam Campground, the pavement ends and the dirt begins. If you've got the

MAP

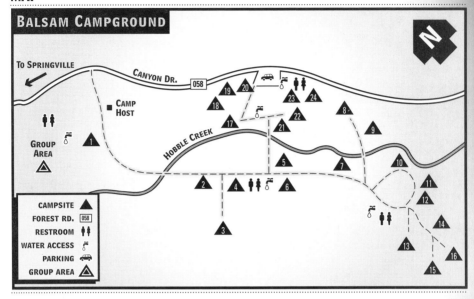

BALSAM CAMPGROUND

To Springville

Canyon Dr. 058

Camp Host

Group Area

Hobble Creek

To Springville

1

19 20
18
17
23 24
22
21
8
9

5
7
10

2
4
6
11
12

3
14

13
16
15

CAMPSITE ▲
FOREST RD. 058
RESTROOM �
WATER ACCESS
PARKING 🚐
GROUP AREA △

---

time, keep going and you'll reach the end of Hobble Creek Canyon and drop into Diamond Fork. The end of pavement also marks the end of camping-restricted areas, so if you're really fixed on the idea of being alone, pull off the dirt road somewhere for dispersed camping and all the solitude you could ever ask for.

Get to Balsam soon, because it won't fly below the radar much longer. Utah's ever-increasing population is constantly seeking new places to explore, and Hobble Creek Canyon just feels like one of those places that's on the cusp of being discovered.

GETTING THERE

From Springville turn east on 400 South, which becomes Canyon Drive and go 13 miles to the campground.

GPS COORDINATES

UTM Zone: 12
Easting: 465772
Northing: 4449872
Latitude: N 40.1985
Longitude: W 111.4022

20
ASPEN GROVE CAMPGROUND

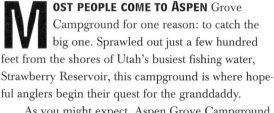

> *This campground is where hopeful anglers begin their quest for the granddaddy.*

MOST PEOPLE COME TO ASPEN Grove Campground for one reason: to catch the big one. Sprawled out just a few hundred feet from the shores of Utah's busiest fishing water, Strawberry Reservoir, this campground is where hopeful anglers begin their quest for the granddaddy.

As you might expect, Aspen Grove Campground sits among a grove of aspen trees on the south side of the Soldier Creek arm of Strawberry Reservoir. The camp is divided between a squatty upper loop and elongated lower line of campsites—53 separate campsites in total. Not every site lives up to its billing as a shaded sanctuary. Here in the Uinta Basin, sagebrush rules the landscape. If the site isn't fortunate enough to have aspens, it's exposed to the wide open landscape of scrubby silvered sage.

To avoid the scrutiny of your neighbors, try for a site in the upper loop. Here, only sites 2, 7, and 16 can be reserved. Sites 12 through 14 are set aside for tents only. It's hit or miss for shade, but you can investigate firsthand. In addition, most sites accommodate RVs, although you'll find less here than at other campgrounds surrounding the reservoir. Besides, the convenience of staying so close to the water is worth having metal-tented neighbors.

If you decide to make reservations (probably a very wise idea on a weekend), take any site from 47 through 52 on the lower string. Venture above or below that magic range, and you'll be left treeless and out in the open. Also, don't go crazy looking for sites 24 through 30. They just don't exist.

Strawberry Reservoir has an interesting past. It was originally built in 1922 as part of the Bureau of Reclamation's Central Utah Project, a boondoggle of water development projects designed to bring water down to the Wasatch Front. In 1973 Strawberry Reservoir was

RATINGS

Beauty: ✩ ✩ ✩ ✩
Privacy: ✩ ✩ ✩
Spaciousness: ✩ ✩ ✩
Quiet: ✩ ✩ ✩
Security: ✩ ✩ ✩
Cleanliness: ✩ ✩ ✩ ✩

enlarged by building Soldier Creek Dam, and now the entire impoundment holds an impressive 1.1 million acre-feet of water (about 360.5 billion gallons).

Because of its size and location, it has always produced large rainbow and cutthroat trout. Unfortunately, nongame species like suckers and chubs have also flourished. In 1990 chubs were doing *too well;* they had taken over and squeezed out most of the trout. The entire reservoir was poisoned and replanted with rainbow and cutthroat trout, as well as kokanee salmon.

Special regulations, including the immediate release of all cutthroat between 15 and 22 inches, are now in place to help keep the chubs in line. As a result, bigger and bigger fish are being caught from Strawberry. There are few other places in Utah one can go (Flaming Gorge, Lake Powell) to consistently catch such sizable fish.

During hot summer months, the fish go to deep waters. Shore fishermen may still find limited success in early morning, but float tubers and boaters net the most fish from about July through the beginning of September. Late fall finds the fish moving in to shallower water, so October may be a good time to stay in Aspen Grove. Unfortunately, bad weather can close the campground before then, although there is some effort made to keep it open through hunting season, when the campground and surrounding area are very popular for the camo-and-blaze crowd. Call ahead to check the campground status.

Strawberry's absolute best fishing is had when the ice comes off the water in the spring. Again, the campground is almost certain to be closed at this point, but it's at least worth investigating.

Just a few hundred yards from the campground is a small boat ramp, complete with ample parking and a small fish-cleaning station. The boat ramp is considerably less crowded than the Strawberry Marina on the reservoir's west side, so don't shy away from the area if you have an aversion to large crowds; you may not feel like you're having a "wilderness experience," but there are certainly more hoppin' places on Strawberry that you could be.

KEY INFORMATION

ADDRESS:	Uinta National Forest Heber Ranger District 2460 South US 40 Heber City, UT 84032
OPERATED BY:	American Land and Leisure
INFORMATION:	(435) 654-0470; www.fs.fed.us/r4/uinta
OPEN:	May–September
SITES:	53
EACH SITE HAS:	Picnic table, fire pit
ASSIGNMENT:	First come, first served; reservations accepted
REGISTRATION:	Self-register on-site; reserve online at www.reserveamerica.com or call (877) 444-6777
FACILITIES:	Flush toilets, drinking water, boat ramp, fish-cleaning station
PARKING:	At campsite only
FEE:	$14 per night single, $28 double; $5 extra vehicle
ELEVATION:	7,670 feet
RESTRICTIONS:	*Fires:* In rings only *Other:* 14-day stay limit

MAP

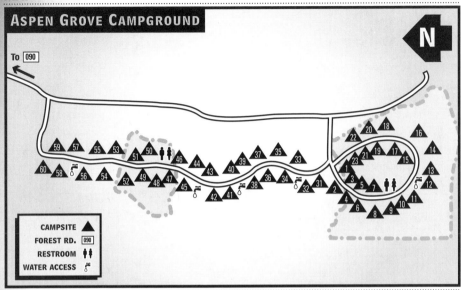

ASPEN GROVE CAMPGROUND

N

To 090

CAMPSITE ▲
FOREST RD. 090
RESTROOM ♀♂
WATER ACCESS

GETTING THERE

From Heber City, go southeast approximately 35 miles on US 40. Turn right on Forest Service Road 090 toward Soldier Creek Dam and continue 5 miles to the campground.

Parents appreciate Aspen Grove campground for its family-friendly setup. Modern restrooms and the availability of drinking water make it a good choice for campers with young ones, and even the most impatient little angler can usually pull in a decent-size trout by floating a worm beneath a bobber at sunup.

If fishing isn't your thing, you may have come to the wrong place. The reservoir's south side is probably the best place to go exploring, but your immediate options are limited due to private property. Then again, if you're just content to be outdoors and don't mind lounging around camp, the convenience of Aspen Grove will suit you just fine.

GPS COORDINATES

UTM Zone: 12
Easting: 496914
Northing: 4441750
Latitude: N 40.1261
Longitude: W 111.0362

21
DRY CANYON CAMPGROUND

THE BRIDGE OVER **D**IAMOND **F**ORK **C**REEK
at Dry Canyon Campground is bigger than is
really necessary. The creek, after all, manages
to ripple but not often splash. Still, it's a perfect frame
for the small river.

Besides its obvious purpose as a means to cross
the river, the bridge serves another, perhaps more
noble mission. It is the only way to access Dry Canyon
Campground. All vehicles must stop and park at the
group parking lot just off of the Diamond Fork
Canyon's main road. Then, campers with their gear in
hand (or on shoulder, strapped to back, or on head)
must walk over the bridge and select their campsite.

It's only a few dozen paces, but something magical
happens when people have to park and walk in to a
campsite. When people leave their AM/FM, CDs,
MP3s, and other advanced technologies behind, they
also seem to leave behind their technological mental
concerns. "I wonder how long it will take us to restruc-
ture the accounting department," turns into, "I wonder
how long it will take me to burn this stick." It's miracu-
lous. And it happens all the time at Dry Canyon.

Dry Canyon Campground is located about 10
miles up Diamond Fork Canyon—a smaller side rift in
the larger and busier Spanish Fork Canyon. Spanish
Fork Canyon hosts the reasonably busy US 89, which
splits to send eastbounders to Green River and Interstate 70, and southbounders all the way to Arizona.

Diamond Fork Canyon's walls parallel the waters
of Diamond Fork Creek, a subdued little stream that
flows downhill until it reaches the Spanish Fork River
along US 89. It's in a shady section of the canyon,
mostly oak trees, after the pavement ends and a well-
maintained dirt road climbs to the upper segment.

Although they're not labeled at camp, I've put
numbers on the map to identify the campsites at Dry

> *Something magical happens when people have to park and walk into a campsite.*

RATINGS
Beauty: ☆ ☆ ☆
Privacy: ☆ ☆ ☆ ☆
Spaciousness: ☆ ☆ ☆ ☆
Quiet: ☆ ☆ ☆ ☆
Security: ☆ ☆ ☆ ☆
Cleanliness: ☆ ☆ ☆ ☆

ADDRESS:	Uinta National Forest Spanish Fork Ranger District 44 West 400 North Spanish Fork, UT 84660
OPERATED BY:	Uinta National Forest
INFORMATION:	(801) 798-3571; www.fs.fed.us/r4/ uinta
OPEN:	May–October
SITES:	6
EACH SITE HAS:	Picnic table, fire ring, barbecue stand
ASSIGNMENT:	First come, first served
REGISTRATION:	None
FACILITIES:	Vault toilets
PARKING:	Group parking
FEE:	None
ELEVATION:	5,479 feet
RESTRICTIONS:	None

Canyon. There are six total, each one hugging the shores of Diamond Fork Creek. The best hugger of the bunch, site 3, is closer to the level ground along the river bed. Sites 1 and 2 sit away and up the hill just a hair, similar to site 6.

You'll have to get creative in sites 4 through 6 when it comes time to put up your tent. There's not a big opening of bare ground, and it's less level than you hope it might be. These sites do sit farthest back from the road, however, so your creativity will be rewarded.

I'm just plain baffled about why there's no fee to camp at Dry Fork. Sure, there's no water. But each site has a nice picnic table and what looks like a new concrete fire ring—amenities that could easily warrant charging a couple of bucks per night.

The most popular hike in the Diamond Fork Canyon begins at the Three Forks Trailhead, less than a mile away from Dry Canyon to the northeast. There are several trails to choose from, but the most well known is the Fifth Water Canyon trail, which leads to the mythical Spanish Fork Canyon hot springs. These hot pools near a spectacular waterfall carry as much anticipation as they do precipitation. They really do exist; you've just got to know how to find them. Park at the trailhead and hike up the river for about a mile before crossing a bridge. Don't cross on the first bridge you see near the trailhead, or you'll never get there. A good online search will give you detailed, step-by-step directions, so do your homework before you go.

Diamond Fork has certainly been picked on lately. It's an important water supply for central Utah, and in recent years the local water conservancy district has installed 6 miles of pipe—the kind big enough to walk through—in a massive construction project. If you see the scars on the landscape, you'll know what they are. Camping along Diamond Fork has been restricted to allow the affected areas to rehabilitate. If you decide not to stay at Dry Canyon on your next trip to Diamond Fork Canyon, check with the Forest Service to see if restrictions have been eased.

In 2006 a large portion of Diamond Fork Creek was poisoned and all fish life was wiped out. It wasn't a chemical spill or toxic waste being dumped into the

MAP

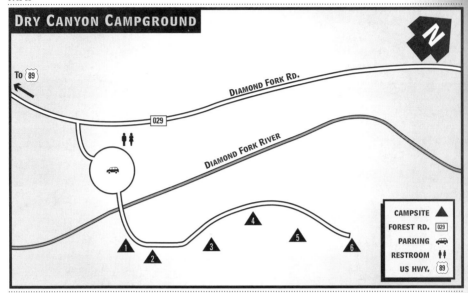

DRY CANYON CAMPGROUND

To 89

DIAMOND FORK RD.

029

DIAMOND FORK RIVER

4

1

2

3

5

6

CAMPSITE	▲
FOREST RD.	029
PARKING	🚗
RESTROOM	🚹🚺
US HWY.	89

river by an unscrupulous company. Rather, Utah's Department of Wildlife Resources made it a goal to remove all species of fish competitive to Bonneville cutthroats and then restock the river with just the Bonnies. Their hope, besides making a unique fishing stream, was to create a permanent home for the disappearing strain of cutthroat and keep it off the federal Threatened or Endangered Species list.

It's unclear what the future of Diamond Fork Creek holds. Its management practices, regulations, and personality as a trout stream are big question marks. Frankly, that's pretty exciting. Those who think they've already done Diamond Fork have the opportunity to rediscover an entirely new place. Newcomers will be able to boast that they were there when the "new" Diamond Fork was born, and can help shape the future of the river and the canyon by telling the Forest Service and other agencies what's working, what's not, and what they'd like to see happen.

For whatever reason, the Forest Service isn't charging a fee to camp at Dry Canyon—at least for now. It would be a bargain at twice the cost (heck, even ten times the cost!) and hopefully it stays that way.

GETTING THERE

From Spanish Fork, go 9 miles east on US 89 and turn left on Forest Service Road 029 (Diamond Fork Road). Go 9 miles up the canyon to the campground.

GPS COORDINATES

UTM Zone: 12

Easting: 468954

Northing: 4436663

Latitude: N 40.0797

Longitude: W 111.3641

22
PONDEROSA CAMPGROUND

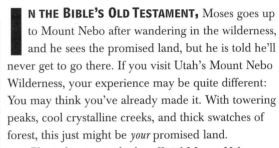

> *With towering peaks, cool crystalline creeks, and thick swatches of forest, this just might be* your *promised land.*

IN THE BIBLE'S OLD TESTAMENT, Moses goes up to Mount Nebo after wandering in the wilderness, and he sees the promised land, but he is told he'll never get to go there. If you visit Utah's Mount Nebo Wilderness, your experience may be quite different: You may think you've already made it. With towering peaks, cool crystalline creeks, and thick swatches of forest, this just might be *your* promised land.

Planted just outside the official Mount Nebo Wilderness boundary is Ponderosa Campground and its 23 campsites. I hope I look as good at age 75 as Ponderosa does, although it's obvious this campground has had some work done. The picnic tables and fire rings are now cast in cement, but the traditional square of cement has been forgone in favor of more organic, rounded shapes that soften the look and complement the curves of Mother Nature. A small sign pays homage to the "visionary men" who planted ponderosa pines here in 1914, almost 20 years before an official campground was constructed in 1933.

The ponderosa pines give this campground not only its name, but also its personality. Their tall, slender trunks shoot up out of an otherwise scrubby landscape. At their feet, the ground is littered with pine needles and the occasional grassy patch, but it remains remarkably flat and even, so you won't have to worry about setting up your tent on a slope and waking up nose to nose with your tent buddy. Beyond the campground in both directions, the plant life is a little more typical of what you might find at this elevation—thick brush, oak, and the occasional lonely evergreen.

Ponderosa pines are great for shade but don't do a great job at providing privacy. They're typically branchless from at least eye level down, so there's no solid shield between you and your neighbors. Fortunately, these individual sites aren't stacked right on top

RATINGS

Beauty: ✿ ✿ ✿ ✿
Privacy: ✿ ✿ ✿
Spaciousness: ✿ ✿ ✿
Quiet: ✿ ✿ ✿ ✿
Security: ✿ ✿ ✿ ✿
Cleanliness: ✿ ✿ ✿

of each other. Pick the right site, position your tent just so, and you'll find enough privacy to get by.

Two-thirds of the sites here can be reserved ahead of time, while sites 1, 5, 7 through 10, 17, and 21 are offered on a first-come, first-served basis. Of the reservables, site 6 offers the most space and backs up into Salt Creek to drown out any unwanted noise. If you're rolling the dice and plan on just showing up to look for a site, try site 8 for all the same reasons as site 6. Both happen to be on the right loop of the campground, but there's nothing wrong with exploring the left loop, which holds sites 14 through 23.

Not too many people spend the night in one of the Nebo Loop area campgrounds, but plenty of Utahns drive the area during the day, especially in the fall. Nebo Loop Road (Forest Service Road 015/048, more commonly called "The Nebo Loop") is arguably Utah's most famous byway for viewing fall foliage. The 32-mile stretch of paved road lifts drivers to more than 9,000 feet in elevation and passes giant groves of maple, oak, and aspen that are woven together in the heart of this section of the Uinta National Forest. Each fall they ignite into a spectacular show of pure reds, brilliant yellows, creamy oranges, and every shade and mixture in between. The Nebo Loop also shows off the dark blue waters of the Payson Lakes (an incredible but crowded camping area), Devil's Kitchen (think baby Bryce Canyon), and breathtaking views of the valley below. If you take the drive, set aside the entire day. You'll want to stop often for photo ops.

Don't shy away from Ponderosa for fear of long lines of loud cars. The beauty of this campground is that it's located on a small spur of FS 048 away from the main Nebo Loop Road. The most traffic you'll see is the more serious outdoors crowd headed for the hiking near the campground.

Just a mile farther up the road is the Andrews Ridge Trailhead. Catch Trail 117 (Nebo Bench) for a rigorous and demanding trek to the top of Nebo Peak. Considering the trailhead sits at around 6,500 feet and the peak about a hundred feet shy of 12,000, you're in for quite a hike. Signage pins the one-way ascent at

KEY INFORMATION

ADDRESS:	Uinta National Forest Spanish Fork Ranger District 44 West 400 North Spanish Fork, UT 84660
OPERATED BY:	American Land and Leisure
INFORMATION:	(801) 798-3571; www.fs.fed.us/r4/ uinta
OPEN:	May–October
SITES:	23
EACH SITE HAS:	Picnic table, fire ring
ASSIGNMENT:	First come, first served; reservations accepted
REGISTRATION:	Self-register on-site; reserve online at www.reserveusa .com or call (877) 444-6777
FACILITIES:	Vault toilets, drinking water
PARKING:	At campsite only
FEE:	$11 per night, $5 day use
ELEVATION:	6,203 feet
RESTRICTIONS:	16-day stay limit

THE BEST
IN TENT
CAMPING
UTAH

MAP

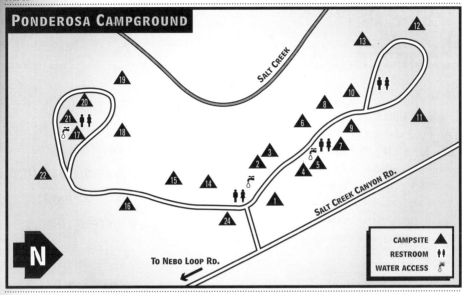

PONDEROSA CAMPGROUND

SALT CREEK

SALT CREEK CANYON RD.

TO NEBO LOOP RD.

N

CAMPSITE
RESTROOM
WATER ACCESS

GETTING THERE

From Nephi, go 6 miles east
on UT 132 to Nebo Loop
Road/FS 048 and turn left.
Go 3.5 miles and stay left
at the fork, then continue
about a half mile to the
campground.

8 miles, although you'll catch Trail 116 (Nebo Peak) for
the last mile and a half. Note that Nebo Peak is different from Mt. Nebo. The two sit about a mile away
from each other, but there's no official trail to connect
them. This is steep and treacherous territory, so use
caution along the trail.

If that seems a little too much, there are plenty of
other trails in and around the Mount Nebo Wilderness
Area, including easier routes to the peak. Check the
Uinta National Forest Web site for excellent route
descriptions as well as maps that include GPS coordinates to help find a trail that suits your needs.

GPS COORDINATES

UTM Zone: 12
Easting: 438836
Northing: 4402277
Latitude: N 39.76823
Longitude: W 111.71413

23
FORKS OF HUNTINGTON CAMPGROUND

A CHAIN OF CAMPSITES DOTS THE LEFT FORK of Huntington Creek just a few hundred feet from the spot where it enters the main creek. A small road leaves the main highway and drops down suddenly to the river's elevation, thick with heavy brush that drinks daily from the crystal clear mountain river water at Forks of Huntington Campground. The air is always cool, the shade plentiful, and the camping unforgettable.

On any lesser creek, a campground at the fork of a tributary and its mother stream would be special, but on Huntington Creek it's really something significant. Here, at just below 8,000 feet, two very prized trout streams combine their flows and create a dilemma for the serious fisherman: Which fork do I fish? In fact, the left, main, *and* right forks of the Huntington are all Blue Ribbon Fisheries.

Stay at Forks of Huntington while you're trying to devise a way to pick your favorite river and you'll be in perfect striking distance of all three. You'll be plenty comfortable—especially if you came with friends. Site 1 is a group site that holds you and up to 49 of your nearest and dearest. Then the camp road rambles up the river to sites 2 and 3, which are set right next to each other and share a water spigot. Another trip up the road puts you at sites 4 and 5, also next-door neighbors. The camp road ends in a small loop with a restroom and the loner of the group, site 6. This is the most private of the sites, spacing-wise, but it doesn't offer much cover from the road and visitors on their way to the restroom. Still, it's probably the site of choice.

Limited in crowd capacity due to its small size, this campground is a better choice than its bigger neighbors. The only downside is, the canyon's best attractions are accessed right along the left fork. That means you'll probably see a lot more of the day-use

> *The air is always cool, the shade plentiful, and the camping unforgettable.*

RATINGS

Beauty: ✪ ✪ ✪ ✪
Privacy: ✪ ✪ ✪
Spaciousness: ✪ ✪ ✪
Quiet: ✪ ✪ ✪
Security: ✪ ✪ ✪ ✪
Cleanliness: ✪ ✪ ✪ ✪

KEY INFORMATION

ADDRESS: Manti-La Sal
National Forest
Ferron/Price Ranger
District
115 West Canyon
Road
Ferron, UT 84523

OPERATED BY: United Land
Management

INFORMATION: (435) 637-2817;
www.fs.fed.us/r4/
mantilasal

OPEN: May–October

SITES: 6

EACH SITE HAS: Picnic table, fire pit

ASSIGNMENT: First come, first
served

REGISTRATION: Self-register on-site

FACILITIES: Vault toilets, water

PARKING: At campsite only

FEE: $8 per night, $4
extra vehicle

ELEVATION: 7,600 feet

RESTRICTIONS: *Pets:* Leashed

crowd breezing in and out of camp. Just keep your valuables locked up tight enough to keep the honest people honest. Don't worry, they go away at night and leave you alone with your bright starry sky.

With any lesser campground, a nearby hiking trail would be a great bonus, but at Forks of Huntington it's something to write home about. This isn't just *any* trail, it's the left fork of Huntington Canyon National Recreation Trail. It's a simple connect-the-dots hike; it links Forks of Huntington Campground and Miller Flat Reservoir. The 4-mile stretch that starts at Forks of Huntington was designated as a National Recreation Trail in 1979, and for good reason. Scattered between the choice fishing pools are several small but scenic waterfalls. A simple snapshot of each one would make a spiffy little screen saver. Take your time behind the camera and you could have a print that's worthy of a real fancy frame.

There are other worthy trails in this part of Manti-La Sal. Go to the Stuart Visitor Information center, a few miles farther up UT 31, to learn about the different trails in the area like Pole Canyon, Short Canyon, or a longer march through the Castle Valley Range.

An informational placard near the bathroom and parking area displays a map with highlighted hiking trails and a chart that briefly describes each hike and ranks its difficulty. No matter which hike you choose, be prepared. The weather is known to turn cold quickly in these canyons, especially as winter approaches.

You may notice several small turnouts along UT 31. Some may indicate that an area is off limits to camping, but most proudly proclaim, "The fee you pay stays here," and then spells out a $3 per vehicle camping charge. These sites aren't anything glamorous—not much more than a scratch in the dirt, a fire ring, and no restrooms. However, they will suffice if Forks of Huntington is full. You'll miss the sounds of a river running by your tent, especially as traffic zips by on the highway, but you won't have any neighbors.

You've already got your fishing pole, so head to Huntington Reservoir, Cleveland Reservoir, or Electric Lake; all located along UT 31. They're all excellent choices to get a taste of alpine fishing without having

MAP

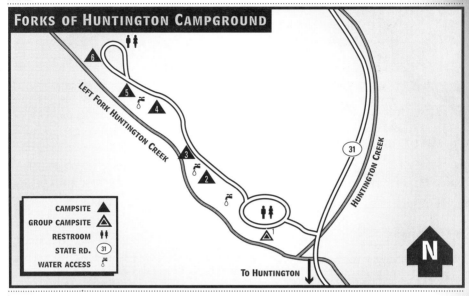

FORKS OF HUNTINGTON CAMPGROUND

LEFT FORK HUNTINGTON CREEK

HUNTINGTON CREEK

31

TO HUNTINGTON

N

CAMPSITE ▲
GROUP CAMPSITE △
RESTROOM ♛♛
STATE RD. ㉛
WATER ACCESS

to hike in. Huntington has been kicking out some pretty beefy tiger trout lately and is a good choice for kids who want to cast from shore. Fishing conditions change throughout the year, but the go-to bait in these parts is a night crawler or minnow suspended beneath a clear bubble.

GETTING THERE

From Huntington, travel 18 miles northwest on UT 31.

GPS COORDINATES

UTM Zone: 12
Easting: 486434
Northing: 4372345
Latitude: N 39.5006
Longitude: W 111.1578

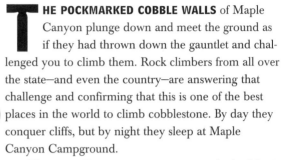

> *Maple Canyon makes rock climbers feel like kids in a candy store.*

THE POCKMARKED COBBLE WALLS of Maple Canyon plunge down and meet the ground as if they had thrown down the gauntlet and challenged you to climb them. Rock climbers from all over the state—and even the country—are answering that challenge and confirming that this is one of the best places in the world to climb cobblestone. By day they conquer cliffs, but by night they sleep at Maple Canyon Campground.

There are 13 sites in a string, just inside the Manti-La Sal National Forest boundary west of the farming town of Moroni. Only one small sign indicates the campground's presence, a brown blur on UT 132 near Fountain Green.

The first of these sites in Maple Canyon is designed to hold groups of up to 40 people. Sites 2 through 4 are individual sites strung along a spur off the main campground road and are probably the best sites in camp, privacy-wise. Because of the high canyon walls, sunshine is at a premium. Sites 5 through 9 give you the most minutes of sunshine each day, which is probably worth considering if you stay here during spring or fall. Sites 10 through 13 are located at the top of the campground, far away from the nine below them.

All of the sites at Maple Canyon can be reserved. If the group site isn't being occupied, it is offered on a first-come, first-served basis at $15 per night. The other sites are also up for grabs when they're not already spoken for, but it only takes a moment to make a reservation, so why risk it?

The restrooms have recently been renovated, which is a welcome improvement from the old ones. They're still vault toilets, but they're sturdy and neat. Water isn't available at camp, but there's a small trickle of a stream that runs adjacent to the road where you

RATINGS

Beauty: ✪ ✪ ✪ ✪
Privacy: ✪ ✪ ✪ ✪
Spaciousness: ✪ ✪ ✪ ✪
Quiet: ✪ ✪ ✪ ✪
Security: ✪ ✪ ✪ ✪ ✪
Cleanliness: ✪ ✪ ✪ ✪

can pump and purify. Bring plenty of your own water in case the stream is dry.

What's not cobbled cliff walls or sandy light brown earth is probably a maple tree. There are a few evergreens to dot the landscape here and there, but most of the green comes from maple trees of every size. For being so close to the Sanpete Valley floor, the canyon is much greener than you'd expect.

Maple Canyon makes rock climbers feel like kids in a candy store. The sheer number and variety of routes available are enough to earn this canyon a reputation as one of the world's best places to climb. An entire book has been written about just this canyon, detailing the different areas to climb, but any gear shop around should be able to point the uninitiated in the right direction.

Difficulty levels range from beginner to hard-core routes for the most insane climbers. Among the most climbed are Engagement Alcove and the Schoolroom, although there are countless climbs known by many names in the area.

Ice climbing is also quite popular in Maple Canyon, but the conditions aren't always favorable. Your best bet would be to hop online and find other climbers in the area who may have a recent report. The campground closes in the wintertime, but ice climbers spend the precious daylight hours tied to the sheer ice walls that form.

Rock climbing isn't the only game in town. Take one of the trails that connect to the side canyons—one to the north and one to the south. They're only short trails that take off right near the campground, but they will give you a hint of the real personality of the canyons of the San Pitch Mountains.

The San Pitch Mountains mark the border between Sanpete and Juab counties. Although they're not too terribly tall, they do rise above the Sanpete Valley and offer convenient camping to residents on both sides. Trails and rough roads snake throughout the range. In fact, it's possible to drive from Wales to Levan on Forest Service Road 101. Find the road by going back out to Westside Road and going south 4 miles to Wales, then turning right. Wales Canyon will lift you up

KEY INFORMATION

ADDRESS:	Manti-La Sal National Forest Sanpete Ranger District 540 North Main Ephraim, UT 84627
OPERATED BY:	Manti-La Sal National Forest
INFORMATION:	(435) 283-4151; www.fs.fed.us/r4/ mantilasal
OPEN:	May–October
SITES:	13
EACH SITE HAS:	Picnic table, fire pit, barbecue stand
ASSIGNMENT:	First come, first served if available; reservations accepted
REGISTRATION:	Reserve online at www.reserveusa. com or call (877) 444-6777
FACILITIES:	Vault toilets
PARKING:	At campsite only
FEE:	$8 per night
ELEVATION:	6,803 feet
RESTRICTIONS:	*Pets:* Leashed *Other:* 14-day stay limit

MAP

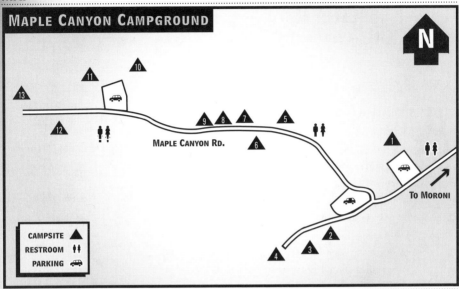

MAPLE CANYON CAMPGROUND

MAPLE CANYON RD.

TO MORONI

CAMPSITE ▲
RESTROOM ♟♟
PARKING 🚗

GETTING THERE

From Moroni, take UT 116
2.5 miles west and turn right
on Westside Road. Go 1.5
miles and turn left on Free-
dom Road, then right on
Maple Canyon Road, past
the turkey farm, 3 miles to
the campground.

over the ridge of the San Pitch Range, then the road
will funnel you back down along Chicken Creek.

I'm not much of a rock climber myself, but I still
found Maple Canyon fascinating. Every texture, every
color, and every little side canyon are so different, yet
they somehow blend together to make it work.

GPS COORDINATES

UTM Zone: 12
Easting: 441031
Northing: 4378706
Latitude: N 39.55601
Longitude: W 111.68640

25
BOWERY CREEK CAMPGROUND

A S SUMMERTIME BRINGS HIGH temperatures, Utahns head for higher elevations. For years, outdoors enthusiasts and heat refugees alike have come to Fish Lake for its crisp air and chilly waters. There are 41 campsites at Bowery Creek that welcome them each season with simple accommodations and a perfect location just minutes from the lake's shore.

There's no easy way to describe the configuration of this campground. There are two access points along the main road, which arc into a diamondlike loop and sprout a triangle zigzag with a baby pyramid at one end and a circle at the other. Ah yes, it's the classic arched-diamond-ziggy-triangasphere. At any rate, the layout makes its way up a hillside away from the lake and road, with a few choice views of the lake valley from scattered breaks in the aspen cover.

If that's your preference—views—try to snatch up site 41 or 42. These two sites, along with 26 others at Bowery Creek, are offered on a first-come, first-served basis. You'd better be one of the first to arrive, because this campground will fill up every weekend all summer long. Sites 32 and 33 are designated for tenters only, and while they're OK options, you'll probably find a more comfy spot elsewhere on the triangasphere—that is, if you don't mind the possibility of spending the night next to a Winnebago. Many of the sites are conducive to RVs, but tents can also occupy the campground.

Reservations are accepted for nine of the individual sites, three double sites, and for three singles. Consider booking one of the larger camps for an extended camping trip or family affair. This is a great place to baptize your outdoors-averse family members into the wonderful world of tall trees and open air. There are modern restrooms at camp and convenience-store concessions available at the nearby Fish Lake Lodge.

> *Baptize your outdoors-averse family members into the wonderful world of tall trees and open air.*

RATINGS

Beauty: ✿ ✿ ✿ ✿
Privacy: ✿ ✿ ✿ ✿
Spaciousness: ✿ ✿ ✿
Quiet: ✿ ✿ ✿
Security: ✿ ✿ ✿
Cleanliness: ✿ ✿ ✿ ✿

KEY INFORMATION

ADDRESS: Fishlake National Forest
Fremont River Ranger District
138 South Main Street
Loa, UT 84747

OPERATED BY: High Country Recreation

INFORMATION: (435) 836-2800; www.fs.fed.us/r4/ fishlake

OPEN: May–September

SITES: 41

EACH SITE HAS: Picnic table, fire pit, barbecue grill

ASSIGNMENT: First come, first served; reservations accepted

REGISTRATION: Self-registration on-site; reserve online at www.reserve usa.com or call (877) 444-6777

FACILITIES: Flush toilets, drinking water

PARKING: At campsite only

FEE: $12 single, $24 double, $36 triple; 50% extra vehicle cost

ELEVATION: 8,892 feet

RESTRICTIONS: *Pets:* Leashed
Other: 10-day stay limit

The sky's the limit around Fish Lake. There are as many things to do there as there are days of the summer. The most obvious attraction is to grab your fishing rod and help the lake live up to its name. Fishing is a big draw here, both in summer when the campgrounds are full, and in winter when they're all closed up. The lake is Utah's biggest natural mountain lake, so it grows some nice-size lake trout. You could dedicate a lifetime to trying to figure out how to land these big boys, but the Forest Service has tried to shave a few years off that endeavor. They offer a contour map of the lake, month-by-month temperature and depth guides, and even suggested lures and techniques on their Web site. Just select "Recreational Activities" from the forest's main Web page, and follow the "Fishing Information" links. Lake trout have company. Browns, rainbows, splake, and perch also swim these waters.

Not enough big fish? Nearby Johnson Valley Reservoir, located just a few miles northeast of Fish Lake along UT 25 is planted with tiger musky, a sterile hybrid of muskellunge and northern pike. These toothy critters are lean, mean eating machines. Currently, you can't even keep a tiger musky at Johnson Valley unless it's more than 40 inches long.

Bring your mountain bike on this camp and choose from several popular trails. If you've got the time, the Mytoge Mountain trail will take you on a 25-mile loop around the entire lake. It's no pedal in the park, however. There are a few climbs that will have you digging deep, and a steep downhill section that requires some delicate maneuvering. Give yourself four or five hours, depending on your condition. Bring lots of water, or even better, pack a lunch. Find the trailhead at the Fish Lake lodge.

The Fishlake National Forest is peppered with little lakes and high mountain streams, which receive only light to moderate recreational use. Forest Service Road 640 (Gooseberry Fremont Road) wanders through some of this territory, eventually passing Gooseberry Campground and connecting with Interstate 70. Gooseberry Campground, not to be confused with the Gooseberry in Manti-La Sal National Forest,

MAP

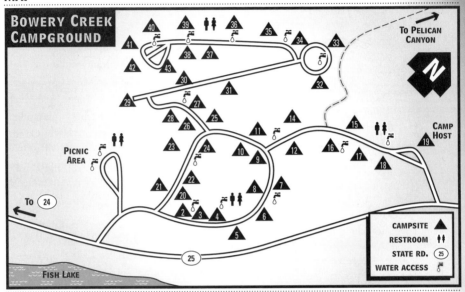

BOWERY CREEK CAMPGROUND

To Pelican Canyon

Camp Host

Picnic Area

To 24

Fish Lake

CAMPSITE	▲
RESTROOM	♀♂
STATE RD.	25
WATER ACCESS	👣

GETTING THERE

From the Junction of UT 24 and UT 25, go northeast 10 miles to the campground.

looks more like a summer camp with its bunkhouses, meeting hall, restrooms, and picnic area, and is the busiest spot on this road. But side roads like Forest Service Road 040 to Rex Reservoir, Forest Service Road 350 to Lost Creek Reservoir, or the trails leaving from Gooseberry will give you more than enough hiking and sightseeing options.

True, the resort atmosphere at Fish Lake does make it hard to feel like you're really roughing it, but once you've ducked back into the campground, climbed into your tent, and pulled your sleeping bag tight up to your chin, you forget all that and just listen to the sounds of nature as they lull you to sleep.

GPS COORDINATES

UTM Zone: 12
Easting: 438395
Northing: 4268448
Latitude: N 38.56234
Longitude: W 111.70710

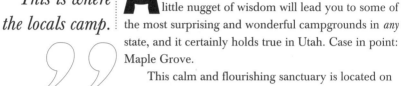

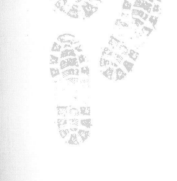

> *This is where the locals camp.*

All great campgrounds can be found in the same place: the last place you'd look for them. This little nugget of wisdom will lead you to some of the most surprising and wonderful campgrounds in *any* state, and it certainly holds true in Utah. Case in point: Maple Grove.

This calm and flourishing sanctuary is located on the foothills of the Pahvant Range between Scipio and Aurora. Don't feel bad if you're not sure where any of those places are, because not many people do. Fish Lake seems to get all the publicity in Fishlake National Forest (gee, I wonder why?), so the Pahvant Range, Tushar Mountains, and Sevier Plateau stay blissfully unadvertised. There are a handful of campgrounds in these parts of Fishlake just like Maple Grove—relatively unknown and unspoiled.

Maple Grove has two parts: first, the main loop with individual sites 1 through 14, and second, three piggybacking loops with group sites A through C. The main loop is separated from the group sites by lovely little Ivy (sometimes noted as "Ivie") Creek, which begins right there in camp by site 14 as it bubbles up from the ground and gurgles its way down the hillside.

Each site is well spaced with good access to one of three spigots on the loop, but be prepared to do a little extra walking every time you need to use the potty if you stay along the back of the loop (sites 5 through 11 or so). Long distance potty-trot or not, numbers 7 and 9 are appropriated a bit more space and privacy than their neighbors. The incontinent can take site 1—also private and very near the restroom.

I asked the campground host there to describe the typical Maple Grove guest. Without hesitation, he replied, "Locals. This is where the locals camp."

I wondered about just *who* was "local" to this locale. Scipio isn't exactly downtown New York, but I

RATINGS

Beauty: ✪ ✪ ✪ ✪
Privacy: ✪ ✪ ✪ ✪
Spaciousness: ✪ ✪ ✪ ✪
Quiet: ✪ ✪ ✪ ✪
Security: ✪ ✪ ✪ ✪
Cleanliness: ✪ ✪ ✪ ✪ ✪

understood what the host was trying to say. This is one of those campgrounds that isn't really a stopping point on the way *to* anywhere, nor a famous destination itself. When the locals want to get out for some peace and quiet, this is where they come. And why not? The canopy created by the maples creates a protective shell against the outside world. And along US 50, there's not a lot of outside world knocking at the door.

The locals have taken good care of Maple Grove; it's in excellent condition. The tables show little sign of use and the trees and bushes surrounding the campsite are in pretty good shape. The graveled road is in great condition and makes this campground accessible to just about anyone. That does include RVs; nearly every site's driveway can accommodate them. I wouldn't worry too much about noise, though. Respect extends beyond the maintenance of the grounds to the treatment of your neighbor. Hopefully that trend continues.

Ivy Creek is planted a couple of times each year with rainbow and brown trout catchables, mostly for the kids during the summer months. They get pretty wily pretty quick, so don't think you're going to have any easy hookups with unwitting hatchery fish. Just be patient—that's the happy fisherman's motto.

Ivy Creek creates a spectacular cascading waterfall about a quarter of a mile back down Maple Grove Road that you'd kick yourself for missing. Pull off toward the river about the time you see an open area with tire tracks on the north side of the road. Just beyond the trees and top lip of the river embankment there's a small trail down to the river below the gorgeous cascade. You're pushing the boundaries of Forest Service property, so watch for posted "No Trespassing" signs.

Bring your camera to capture this magnificent display of tumbling water. Rather than one forceful plunge, the watery fingers of these falls crawl between rocks and over lush green grasses before tumbling down to small pools, collecting, and slowly moving back down to the valley floor. It's mesmerizing.

There are many campers who come to Maple Grove to access the Paiute ATV trail, which traverses

ADDRESS:	**Fishlake National Forest Fillmore Ranger District 390 South Main Street Fillmore, UT 84631**
OPERATED BY:	**Fishlake National Forest**
INFORMATION:	**(435) 743-5721; www.fs.fed.us/r4/ fishlake**
OPEN:	**May–October**
SITES:	**20 plus 3 group sites**
EACH SITE HAS:	**Picnic table, fire pit, barbecue stand**
ASSIGNMENT:	**First come, first served**
REGISTRATION:	**Self-register on-site**
FACILITIES:	**Vault toilets, drinking water**
PARKING:	**At campsite only**
FEE:	**$10 per night; $5 extra vehicle**
ELEVATION:	**6,486 feet**
RESTRICTIONS:	*Pets:* **Leashed** *Other:* **Firewood gathering prohibited**

MAP

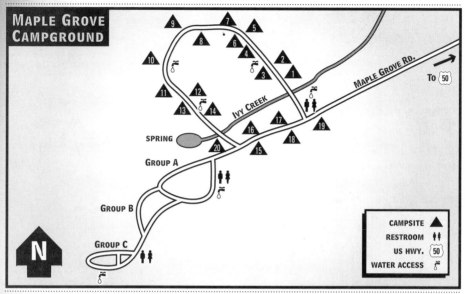

MAPLE GROVE CAMPGROUND

IVY CREEK

MAPLE GROVE RD.

To 50

SPRING

GROUP A

GROUP B

GROUP C

N

CAMPSITE	▲
RESTROOM	♀♂
US HWY.	50
WATER ACCESS	⚲

GETTING THERE

From Scipio, drive 15 miles southeast on US 50, then turn right on Maple Grove Road, following the sign 4 miles to the campground.

a huge chunk of Fishlake National Forest. ATVs are prohibited in the campground, so you won't have to contend with buzzing motors when you're trying to sleep in.

Trails leave from camp and eventually meet back up with Forest Service Road 096. You can take the road north and scale Coffee Peak or south to try Jacks Peak. Both are just over 10,000 feet in elevation and will let you peek over the Pahvant Range to see the Sevier Desert to the west. Frankly, you could wander around exploring side canyons for days, crisscrossing the Paiute trail the whole way through.

GPS COORDINATES

UTM Zone: 12
Easting: 405724
Northing: 4319393
Latitude: N 39.01849
Longitude: W 112.08901

DEEP **CREEK** CAMPGROUND

DEEP **CREEK CAMPGROUND** is one of those off-the-beaten-path campgrounds that makes you question why you ever stick to *any* beaten path. In a region of Utah dominated by big and busy campgrounds in the Flaming Gorge National Recreation Area, Deep Creek exists in its own little bubble, just a few miles away on the north slope of the Uinta Mountains.

> *Deep Creek exists in its own little bubble.*

This serene little campground is a short string of sites with a small needle's-eye loop on the back side. Sites 1 through 4 are found at the campground entrance and offer two of the best sites in camp, 2 and 4. The campground road then passes a small bridge over the trickling waters of Deep Creek to the remaining 13 sites. Sites 5 and 10 will put you closest to the creek, but site 7 is where you're going to find the privacy and convenience of being separated from other campers and close (but not too close) to the bathroom. Site 11 backs up toward a large rock cliff and can give you excellent shade, for at least half the day.

Aspen and Engelmann spruce make a patchwork of tree cover, while the waters of Deep Creek and frequent afternoon rainstorms provide plenty of precipitation for prolific brush, especially at the creek's edges. Be conscientious of the riparian habitat and the deadfall in the creek. Campers seeking firewood gutted the creek over time and unwittingly impaired much of the fish habitat, so the Forest Service placed logs and other deadfall back into the river to help restore it to health in 2004.

In fact, if there's one complaint to be had for Deep Creek, it's the obvious mistreatment it's had from campers over the years. The sites here just didn't feel orderly—an old clothesline in site 10, broken limbs in many trees. A campground can't help but show wear, but it shouldn't have tear. Indeed this campground is well used and will probably fill right up on

RATINGS

Beauty: ✩ ✩ ✩ ✩
Privacy: ✩ ✩ ✩ ✩
Spaciousness: ✩ ✩ ✩ ✩ ✩
Quiet: ✩ ✩ ✩ ✩
Security: ✩ ✩ ✩ ✩
Cleanliness: ✩ ✩ ✩

ADDRESS: Ashley National
Forest
Flaming Gorge
Ranger District
P.O. Box 279
Manila, UT 84046

OPERATED BY: Flaming Gorge
Corp.

INFORMATION: (435) 784-3445;
www.fs.fed.us/r4/
ashley

OPEN: June 15–
September 15

SITES: 17

EACH SITE HAS: Picnic table, fire pit

ASSIGNMENT: First come, first
served

REGISTRATION: Self-register on-site

FACILITIES: Vault toilets

PARKING: At campsite only

FEE: $9 per night

ELEVATION: 7,727 feet

RESTRICTIONS: *Pets:* Leashed
Other: 16-day stay
limit

the weekends, but its out-of-the-way location should only heighten the concern and care for such a nifty little place. Hopefully this renewed attention to the creek will help campers contemplate how special the campground really is.

Fishing opportunities abound in the Uintas, and this is no exception. Deep Creek holds a few small rainbow trout, but for a few more rainbows, slide down to Carter Creek, located just past camp at the terminus of Deep Creek. Carter Creek begins in this region and flows all the way into Flaming Gorge. Sheep Creek is also planted with rainbows. Find this more popular river by continuing on Forest Service Road 539 to Forest Service Road 218 (Sheep Creek Loop), or find paved access on UT 44 back toward Manila at the bottom of Sheep Creek Bay, where it enters the reservoir.

High-mountain lakes dot the Uinta backcountry and almost guarantee the solitude-seeker a chance at catching a pan-sized brook trout. Elk Park trails 013 and 014 (you pass their trailhead on FS 539 on your way to the campground) will eventually lead to some of these opportunities, but in a very roundabout way. These trails are better suited for scenery seekers who won't be disappointed by broad views of Flaming Gorge. Alpine fishermen are better served by driving to Browne Lake or Spirit Lake on Forest Service Road 221 and hiking anywhere from 1 to 8 miles for a choice of 30-plus little lakes.

Most visitors to this part of Daggett County do come for the unparalleled fishing opportunities at Flaming Gorge Reservoir, more commonly referred to as "The Gorge." Monstrous lake trout have given rise to urban legends about dam repairmen refusing to dive without cages due to "car-size fish." While those reports may be exaggerated, the current state record 50-pound lake trout and 33-pound brown trout both came from the Gorge, so there are some brutes. The Green River is also touted as some of the west's best fly-fishing in the stretches just below the dam.

Within an hour's drive of Deep Creek you'll find no fewer than 25 campgrounds, picnic areas, or reservoir access points. This massive body of water and accompanying land area covers around 200,000 acres

MAP

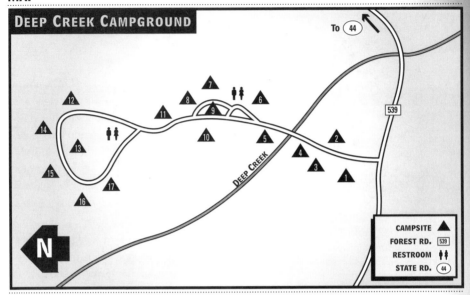

DEEP CREEK CAMPGROUND

To 44

539

CAMPSITE ▲
FOREST RD. 539
RESTROOM ♀♂
STATE RD. 44

DEEP CREEK

N

of designated recreational area, divided almost equally between Utah and Wyoming. While these campgrounds are unique (boat-in only areas, an island), they all have one thing in common—they're usually packed from season's open to season's end. Choose to stay away from the madness. If you decide to go the Gorge, you'll just have to drive a few extra minutes from Deep Creek.

Truth be told, there are several sweet little campgrounds like this one throughout the Uintas. Deep Creek is one of the most accessible and serves as the perfect primer for what this fantastic mountain range has to offer. Do yourself a favor: Avoid the crowds around Flaming Gorge, get off the main roads, and let Deep Creek Campground work its charm on your next camping trip to northeastern Utah.

GETTING THERE

From Manila, go 15 miles south on UT 44, then turn right on FS 539 and go 4 miles to the campground.

GPS COORDINATES

UTM Zone: 12
Easting: 607075
Northing: 4523436
Latitude: N 40.85499
Longitude: W 109.72963

WESTERN UTAH

28

CLEAR CREEK CAMPGROUND

POP QUIZ: How many national forests are there in Utah? Six? Wrong. Seven? Nope. Try eight. Avid outdoorsmen could probably rattle off the first six: Ashley, Dixie, Fishlake, Manti-La Sal, Uinta, and Wasatch-Cache. But Caribou and Sawtooth? Yep. And Sawtooth holds one of Utah's sweet little treasures—Clear Creek Campground.

Like an island surrounded by a sea of unremarkable countryside, Sawtooth National Forest's Raft River Mountain Range is all alone in northwestern Utah. If that doesn't sound so bad—being all alone—then make Clear Creek Campground the top priority on your "to-camp" list. Solitude comes in spades in this cozy little campground.

Clear Creek is truly isolated. There's no fee, no numbers on the campsites, and not much sign that more than a handful of people ever make it here, especially on a weekday. Don't mistake isolation for desolation, though. The campground's namesake, sparkling Clear Creek, makes its way through the camp and gives life to numerous tall aspens and evergreens, with a healthy riparian understory of thick brush along the creek's shores and throughout the camp's gentle hillside. The creek is also rumored to hold small trout for sneak-attack-style fishing, although someone must have given them warning when I came—I never actually saw any myself.

The campsites here are mostly standard—a small fire pit and picnic table on a flat patch of ground. They're not numbered at the campground, but they've been labeled in the map here for reference. You shouldn't have any trouble snagging site 7 or 8 to maximize privacy if there are other campers around. Sites 1 and 2 should be your last pick. Their lack of shade and exposure to the road make them less desirable than others farther down the road. The Forest Service

> *Solitude comes in spades in this cozy little campground.*

RATINGS

Beauty: ✿ ✿ ✿
Privacy: ✿ ✿ ✿ ✿ ✿
Spaciousness: ✿ ✿ ✿ ✿ ✿
Quiet: ✿ ✿ ✿ ✿ ✿
Security: ✿ ✿ ✿ ✿ ✿
Cleanliness: ✿ ✿ ✿ ✿

ADDRESS:	Sawtooth National Forest
	Minidoka Ranger District
	3650 South Overland Avenue
	Burley, ID 83318
OPERATED BY:	Sawtooth National Forest
INFORMATION:	(208) 678-0430; www.fs.fed.us/r4/sawtooth
OPEN:	June–September
SITES:	8
EACH SITE HAS:	Picnic table, fire pit
ASSIGNMENT:	First come, first served
REGISTRATION:	None
FACILITIES:	Vault toilets
PARKING:	At campsite only
FEE:	None
ELEVATION:	6,303 feet
RESTRICTIONS:	*Fires:* In rings only

says there are 14 sites total, but I only found 8. Perhaps the other six were hiding with the fish.

Even though the driving directions sound a bit tricky, getting to the campground is actually easy. Don't panic when you see the "Welcome To Idaho" signs on UT 42. You will briefly enter the Gem State before dipping back into Utah by following the brown recreation signs. The family car will make the well-maintained dirt road just fine, but bring plenty of supplies. Snowville (population 177) is the closest sign of civilization, but you'll have to make it to Brigham City, Utah, or Burley, Idaho, for real supplies. Each is somewhere on the order of an hour and a half away, each way.

There's lots of exploring to be done in the Raft River Range. Most notable are the hikes taken from the Bull Flat Trailhead, located across from site 8 in the back loop of the campground. Take a fork off the main trail after about a mile to go to Bull Flat, or stay on the main trail to climb to beautiful Bull Lake, and then on to the peak of Bull Mountain. Once on top of the summit you'll have staggering views of Utah, Idaho, and Nevada. Considering the campground is at 6,300 feet in elevation and the peak at just less than 10,000, you should be prepared to climb. Take the trail as an overnight backpacking trip to help break up all the steep terrain and give you more time to see the sights.

On the other side of the mountain you may notice a large, cavelike opening etched out of the stone face high on the hilltop. I wouldn't recommend making the trek up there; there's no real trail to the area and it's incredibly steep and rugged. There are, however, remnants of a few old mines if you decide to head off in that direction. Do so at your own risk, and be aware and respectful of the plentiful fences and private property boundaries in the area.

Once you've discovered the Raft River Range, you'll likely want to come back again and again. The Clear Creek and Bull Flat areas only hold a portion of the surprises you might find in this unique little mountain range. Its western reaches also have little canyons with spring-fed streams folded inside.

If you didn't pass the pop quiz, here's your chance to take a field trip to Sawtooth National Forest.

MAP

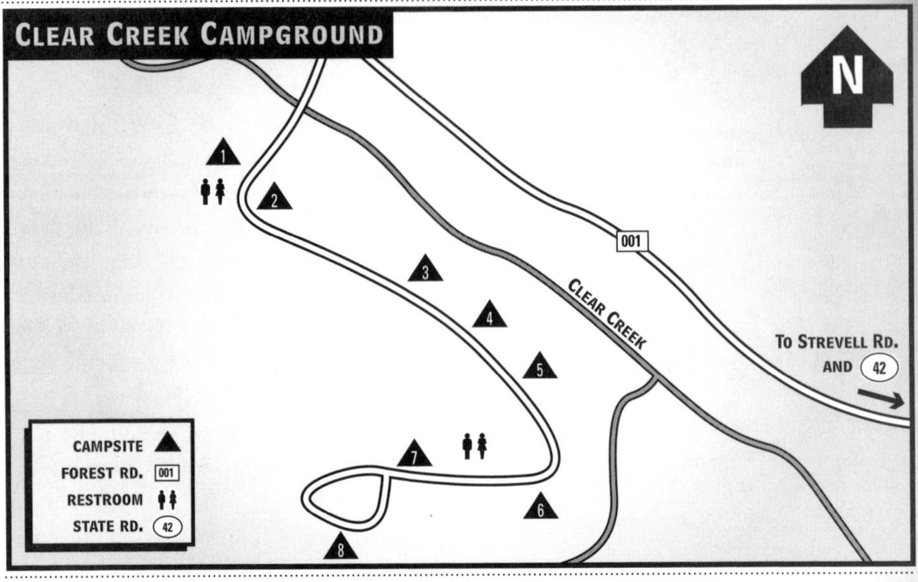
CLEAR CREEK CAMPGROUND
N
001
CLEAR CREEK
TO STREVELL RD. AND 42
1
2
3
4
5
6
7
8
CAMPSITE
FOREST RD. 001
RESTROOM
STATE RD. 42

(Coincidentally, the other seldom-known national forest in Utah—Caribou—has only a dot of land in Utah near Plymouth on the Box Elder/Cache County line. There are no formal campgrounds there, but the Clarkston Mountain's Gunsight Peak looms at 8,244 feet.) While it may not be the biggest or most famous of national forests, Sawtooth holds hidden treasures for the solitude seekers willing to find them.

GETTING THERE

From Snowville, go 26 miles west (becoming northwest) on UT 30 (which becomes UT 42) past Curlew Junction, then turn left on Strevell Road. Take Strevell 3 miles, then turn left (south) on Clear Creek Road (Forest Service Road 001) and continue 6 miles to the campground.

GPS COORDINATES

UTM Zone: 12
Easting: 307468
Northing: 4647230
Latitude: N 41.95356
Longitude: W 113.32301

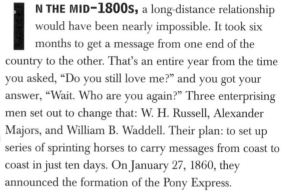

> *The west desert is alive and rich with history, wildlife, and plenty for campers to do.*

IN THE MID-**1800s,** a long-distance relationship would have been nearly impossible. It took six months to get a message from one end of the country to the other. That's an entire year from the time you asked, "Do you still love me?" and you got your answer, "Wait. Who are you again?" Three enterprising men set out to change that: W. H. Russell, Alexander Majors, and William B. Waddell. Their plan: to set up series of sprinting horses to carry messages from coast to coast in just ten days. On January 27, 1860, they announced the formation of the Pony Express.

Simpson Springs, located in Utah's west desert, was an important watering station and rest house for riders along the Pony Express route. Although the Pony Express only operated for less than two years, its heritage has been preserved at Simpson Springs.

A large campground located just off the old Pony Express route is home to 20 smallish sites, each equipped with its own picnic table and not much else. Water is available from several spigots around the campground, but it must be treated before drinking.

So many buildings have been erected, destroyed, replaced, and repaired in the Simpson Springs area that no one quite is sure which building was the original Pony Express station. Today, a small reimagined station stands across the road from the campground as a re-creation of what the original building would have looked like, in what is believed to be the approximate place the original was built. Duck inside the squatty little cabin and try to imagine yourself being a pony rider coming in from his hot, dusty sprint for a little rest and shelter from the sun.

Several interpretive signs are located back toward the parking area, including a brief history that recounts the rise and fall of the Pony Express, as well as the chronicled history of Simpson Springs itself.

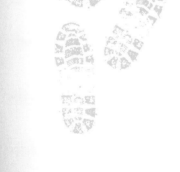

RATINGS

Beauty: ✿ ✿ ✿
Privacy: ✿ ✿
Spaciousness: ✿ ✿ ✿
Quiet: ✿ ✿ ✿ ✿ ✿
Security: ✿ ✿ ✿ ✿ ✿
Cleanliness: ✿ ✿ ✿ ✿ ✿

Summers can be scorching in Utah's west desert, so most people come to Simpson Springs in the cool seasons. If that's your plan, just make sure it hasn't been too wet for the days preceding your trip; the dirt road can get a little slick. Otherwise, your family sedan will make the trip just fine.

If you must travel in summer, try to get site number 1 or number 20 for shade. In cool times, sites 8, 18, or 19 are set a bit back from the others to offer a bit of privacy (though not much) in an otherwise uncovered landscape.

Simpson Springs had a resurgence in the 1940s after the completion of the transcontinental telegraph doomed the Pony Express and let the area lie largely unattended for 80 years. From 1939 to 1942, the Civilian Conservation Corps built barracks, a mess hall, a swimming pool, and other buildings as a base for their range and road operations in the valley. All was torn down at the beginning of World War II, but the foundations and remnants of that development line the road up to the campground.

Simpson Springs has great history, and also hosts a menagerie of Utah's most unique wildlife. Hundreds of pronghorn antelope live in the hills surrounding the old Pony Express Trail, and cross the road each day as they graze in the area. Hawks rule the skies, and if you're really lucky, you may even catch a glimpse of one of the herds of wild horses in the region. The Bureau of Land Management (BLM) manages some 3,000 wild horses and 100 wild burros throughout Utah. I was lucky enough to see about a dozen of these magnificent creatures on my way to the campground. The Wild West indeed!

Continue west nearly 40 miles along the Pony Express Trail to visit Fish Springs National Wildlife Refuge, where you'll encounter a true oasis in the desert. Scores of birds, mammals, reptiles, and even a native fish call this 18,000-acre refuge (10,000-acre marsh) home. Pack your camera to take pictures of some of these species around the refuge; you'll probably need the photos to convince your friends that this place really exists. See **www.fws.gov/fishsprings** for more information.

KEY INFORMATION

ADDRESS:	Bureau of Land Management Salt Lake Field Office 2370 South 2300 West Salt Lake City, UT 84119
OPERATED BY:	Bureau of Land Management
INFORMATION:	(801) 977-4300; www.ut.blm.gov
OPEN:	Year-round
SITES:	20
EACH SITE HAS:	Picnic table, barbecue stand
ASSIGNMENT:	First come, first served
REGISTRATION:	Self-register on-site
FACILITIES:	Vault toilets, water (NON-potable)
PARKING:	At campsite only
FEE:	$5 per night
ELEVATION:	4,890 feet
RESTRICTIONS:	*Other:* 14-day stay limit; woodcutting prohibited

MAP

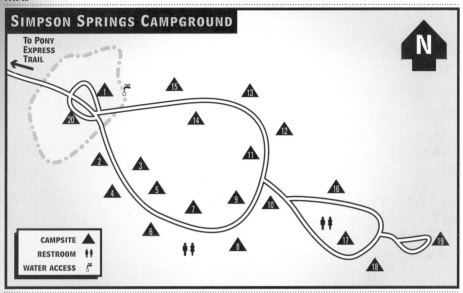

SIMPSON SPRINGS CAMPGROUND

To Pony Express Trail

N

CAMPSITE ▲
RESTROOM 👫
WATER ACCESS 🚰

GETTING THERE

From Vernon, go 5 miles north on UT 36 and turn left on Lookout Pass Road (also labeled as old Pony Express Trail). Go west over Lookout Pass where the road turns to dirt and continue a total of approximately 30 miles, following signs to the campground.

Another 40 miles to the west from Fish Springs is the Deep Creek Mountain Range—a sharp series of peaks that rises dramatically from the flat desert floor. Here you'll find a few small creeks with beautifully colored small trout and a chance to hike the daunting 12,087-foot Ibapah Peak. Most hikers stay at the BLM's rustic CCC campground south of Callao, but you can day trip from Simpson Springs if you don't mind the long drive.

Unbeknownst to most Utahns, the world does not end after the city of Tooele. The west desert is alive and rich with history, wildlife, and plenty for campers to do; and there's no place better to start your discoveries than at Simpson Springs campground.

GPS COORDINATES

UTM Zone: 12
Easting: 347471
Northing: 4433362
Latitude: N 40.03670
Longitude: W 112.78780

LOOP CAMPGROUND

THE LONELY STANSBURY MOUNTAINS can make you feel like you're stranded on an island. You should be so lucky as to be stuck with this mountain range to explore. Surrounded by sand and sage on three sides and the salty waters of the Great Salt Lake to the northeast, the Stansbury Range is a bona fide oasis in the desert.

Loop Campground can't help but earn its name. South Willow Canyon has six separate campgrounds and Loop is the last one on the road. The campground abuts the Deseret Peak Wilderness Area, so the long skinny loop of the campground is created when the road turns to direct cars back down the canyon.

Along the loop are the campsites—average in size and in well-used condition. Within the loop is a smaller circular turnoff where you can access sites 3 through 5. If you can, pick another site besides these. Site number 1, for example, is probably the gem of the campground. It's the first site you'll come to, located at the top of a steep dirt driveway. If you're lucky enough to snag this site, you probably won't see another human being while you're in camp. Sites 1A and 2 are also scattered on the first side of the loop and make for semi-shielded camping.

The biggest disadvantage to camping in Loop is the lack of drinking water, although a nearby stream provides all the water you care to filter, making that problem a non-issue. Old but usable vault toilets are evenly spaced among the sites, and garbage service is available.

The main draw to this part of the Stansbury Range is the Deseret Peak Wilderness Area and the 4-mile (one-way) trail to Deseret Peak. Loop Campground serves as the trailhead for the hike, so there's a small parking area at the top of the loop. If you're in good condition, get up early and take the hike to the

> *Once you visit Loop Campground you'll want to tell everyone about the Stansbury Mountains.*

RATINGS

Beauty: ✪ ✪ ✪ ✪ ✪
Privacy: ✪ ✪ ✪ ✪
Spaciousness: ✪ ✪ ✪ ✪
Quiet: ✪ ✪ ✪ ✪
Security: ✪ ✪ ✪ ✪
Cleanliness: ✪ ✪ ✪ ✪

KEY INFORMATION

ADDRESS: Wasatch-Cache National Forest Salt Lake Ranger District 6944 South 3000 East Salt Lake City, UT 84121

OPERATED BY: American Land and Leisure

INFORMATION: www.fs.fed.us/r4/wcnf/unit/slrd/recreation

OPEN: Late May–mid-October (weather permitting)

SITES: 9

EACH SITE HAS: Picnic table, fire ring

ASSIGNMENT: First come, first served; no reservations

REGISTRATION: Self-register on-site

FACILITIES: Vault toilets, garbage service

PARKING: At campsite only

FEE: $8 per night single sites, $16 per night double site; $5 each additional vehicle

ELEVATION: 7,440 feet

RESTRICTIONS: *Pets:* Leashed
Fires: In rings only
Other: 7-day stay limit; gate closed 10 p.m.–6 a.m.

peak. You'll have to make more than 3,500 feet in elevation, but the 360-degree panorama views are unmatched. From Deseret Peak, look around and you'll see you really are on an island. The Great Basin—miles and miles of nothing—surrounds you. Pack a lunch and enjoy your position on top of the desert while gazing at the rocky outcropping and patchwork of pine and aspen on the canyon floor. Just be sure to head down if there's any sign of a storm. Lightning and bald mountain peaks don't mix well for a hiker. Add in wet rocks on a steep trail and you've got a recipe for one heck of a laceration cocktail.

Deseret Peak isn't the only hike in the 25,000-acre wilderness. Instead of staying on the Mill Fork trail, take the Willow Lakes trail. This trail clings to the hillside and skirts around a couple of valleys before dropping you into South Willow Lake. Climb back out and hug one more ridge to reach North Willow Lake. Just beware of so-called shortcuts. No matter how skilled you think you are, dropping down into one of these valleys to follow the river back to camp is a bad idea, especially in the snow … I've heard.

For some reason, Loop and the other campgrounds of South Willow Canyon aren't used nearly as much as the campgrounds in the Wasatch Range. Perhaps it's the old adage, "Out of sight, out of mind." The Oquirrh Mountains stand between the Salt Lake Valley and the Stansbury Mountains, blocking them from the view of Utah's most populated area. Consequently, you've got a good chance at finding a site at Loop, even when campgrounds in Big and Little Cottonwood Canyons of the Wasatch Range are busting at the seams. The hiking trails here are also in better shape—less litter, less sign of human damage, and more solitude.

Don't mistake "forgotten" for "neglected," though. There is a small ranger station in the canyon and campgrounds are often patrolled. The dedication of the rangers ensures the protection of this precious and rare resource in the desert, but means you need to make doubly sure you're familiar with forest and wilderness regulations before heading out. Mountain bikes and OHVs are often seen in the canyon but are prohibited within the wilderness boundary.

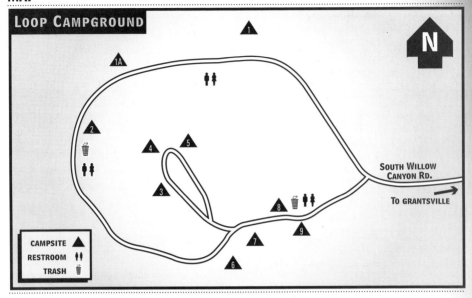

LOOP CAMPGROUND

SOUTH WILLOW CANYON RD.

TO GRANTSVILLE

CAMPSITE ▲
RESTROOM ♂♀
TRASH 🗑

GETTING THERE

Once you visit Loop Campground you'll want to tell everyone about the Stansbury Mountains. Instead of just telling them, why not load them in the car and head out to the desert? Just when they think you've gone nuts, you'll make the turn into South Willow Canyon, leave the pavement, and crawl up to Loop Campground. You'll open their eyes to a sweet little mountain retreat and have a quiet little piece of the island all to yourselves.

From Salt Lake City, take Interstate 80 west 20 miles to Exit 99 (Lake Point/UT 36). Go 3.5 miles south on UT 36, then turn right toward Grantsville on UT 138. Go west on UT 138 for 10 miles, passing through most of Grantsville, then turn left on 400 West at the signed areas for North Willow and South Willow Recreation Areas. Drive south about 5 miles and turn right at the South Willow turnoff. Loop Campground is 13 miles up South Willow Canyon on a paved-then-graveled road.

GPS COORDINATES

UTM Zone: 12
Easting: 363844
Northing: 4482619
Latitude: N 40.48311
Longitude: W 112.60643

> *It's almost hypnotic to stand near the bubbling water.*

Native Americans in the Goshute tribe named it Shambip, early settlers regarded it as their lifeblood, and members of the Civilian Conservation Corps once called it home. Although now it's just known as Clover Springs Campground, it's still relatively unknown as a neat little place to spend the night in your tent.

Because it's only 60 miles from Salt Lake City, you'd expect this 11-site campground to fill up every night with urbanites looking for a quick overnight getaway. On the contrary, that demographic seems to congregate in the canyons of the Wasatch Front, leaving Clover Springs to the locals and the lucky few who have discovered its location.

There are two sections of the campground: sites 1 through 7 where horses are prohibited, and sites 8 through 11 where they are welcome. Upon entering the campground, the division of these two factions is apparent; equestrians go right along a gentle incline to find large hitching rails and watering troughs, and the horseless go left to choose from several sites that sit along the shores of Clover Creek.

Snag site 2, 4, or 6 for the most shade and privacy in the campground. You'll also have the bonus of being sung to sleep at night by the icy cold waters of Clover Creek as they amble by, just feet from each of these sites. The creek is actually born right there in the campground at the springs, located just up from site number 2 at Clover Springs. It's almost hypnotic to stand near the bubbling water as it burps out of the ground and flows away.

The springs have given life to towering cottonwood trees and green grasses in the campsites closest to the water. This burst of green fades into hardy junipers that dot the entire hillside here at the base of the Onaqui Mountains.

RATINGS

Beauty: ✿ ✿ ✿
Privacy: ✿ ✿ ✿
Spaciousness: ✿ ✿ ✿ ✿
Quiet: ✿ ✿ ✿
Security: ✿ ✿ ✿ ✿
Cleanliness: ✿ ✿ ✿ ✿

The equestrian side is decidedly less lush, being removed from the water. If all the lower sites are taken, sites 10 and 11 are actually quite nice, and you won't see much traffic up there at the end of the campground road. They slip under juniper cover and are quite cozy in their own right.

Site number 7 is also worthy of consideration as a group site. It's got ample parking, plenty of shade, and enough seating and serving areas to keep it from feeling crowded. It's a steal at only $25 per night and is the only site in the campground that can be reserved. Call the Bureau of Land Management (BLM) at (801) 977-4300 for more information.

You may be tempted to cup your hands into the waters of Clover Springs and gulp down the spring water, especially in the summer months when this campground sizzles, but campers are warned not to drink the water. Also, the toilets are only small huts, and although they're tidy and functional, you'll definitely know you've left the comforts of your own potty back at home.

Horseback riding is one of the big draws to Clover Springs, but don't feel like you can't explore using your own two legs. The Onaqui Range is more hill than mountain, but it still holds days and days full of exploration. Find seasonal springs, old mines, and cute little canyons littered throughout the range. Flowering cacti dot the landscape, and even the occasional Sego Lily, Utah's official state flower, can be found and photographed. The range peaks out at around 9,000 feet for climbers adamant about finding the best views. Trails are sketchy, but a small trail that introduces you to the area leaves right from camp.

Continue up UT 199 to Johnson Pass for some great views of Utah's west desert to the west and the Oquirrh Mountains back to the east. This area was once buzzing with activity in the mid-1930s as members of the CCC's Company 2517 worked in the area and were based where the Clover Springs Campground now sits. Imagine what these young men might have thought, many of them from the more rain-blessed regions of the eastern United States, as they looked out over Johnson's Pass to Utah's most desolate region.

KEY INFORMATION

ADDRESS:	Bureau of Land Management Salt Lake Field Office 2370 South 2300 West Salt Lake City, UT 84119
OPERATED BY:	Bureau of Land Management
INFORMATION:	(801) 977-4300; www.ut.blm.gov/ recsite/otherpages/ clover.html
OPEN:	May–November
SITES:	11
EACH SITE HAS:	Picnic table, fire ring
ASSIGNMENT:	First come, first served; group site reservable
REGISTRATION:	Self-register on-site
FACILITIES:	Vault toilets
PARKING:	At campsite only
FEE:	$6 per night
ELEVATION:	6,004 feet
RESTRICTIONS:	*Fires:* Check at campground

MAP

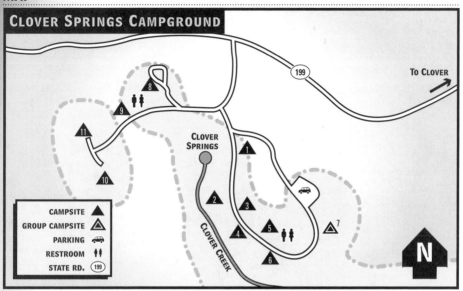

CLOVER SPRINGS CAMPGROUND

199

TO CLOVER

8

9

11

CLOVER
SPRINGS

1

10

2

3

5

4

7

6

N

CLOVER CREEK

CAMPSITE	▲
GROUP CAMPSITE	△
PARKING	🚐
RESTROOM	👫
STATE RD.	199

GETTING THERE

From Tooele, go 16 miles south on UT 36, then turn right on UT 199. Continue 8 miles west on UT 199 to the campground.

GPS COORDINATES

UTM Zone: 12

Easting: 368336

Northing: 4467439

Latitude: N 40.34712

Longitude: W 112.55031

The Onaqui Mountains are sandwiched between two funny little islands of national forest lands: the Deseret Peak complex to the north and the Sheeprock Mountains/Vernon Reservoir complex to the south. Deseret Peak is addressed in the Loop Campground chapter of this book (Campground #30), but the Sheeprock area campground I visited, Indian Creek, didn't make the cut. This was due primarily to the fact that it no longer exists, which made it tough to discuss in any detail, and near impossible to draw on a map. It was still fun to wander around there, and you can do the same by going back out to UT 36 and driving south to Vernon. Follow the signs just past town to Vernon Reservoir, and you'll have access to several dirt roads that wind around those hills.

Clover Springs is open through November, weather permitting. By this time, most other campgrounds in northern Utah are closed, so this is an ideal place to keep in your back pocket for those times in late fall when you're itching to get out but don't have the time to travel to southern Utah. If spring weather has been cooperative, the sites here may be campable earlier than May.

SOUTHERN **UTAH**

32
NATURAL BRIDGES
NATIONAL MONUMENT

SOMEWHERE BETWEEN THE TINY TOWN of Blanding and the recreation hotspot of Lake Powell lies the tiny little desert isle of Natural Bridges National Monument. The park only encompasses 7,636 acres, but each one holds something special that's just begging to be discovered.

Only about 125,000 people visit Natural Bridges each year, so the campground within the park is actually a great place to spend the night. That might seem like a lot of visitors, but consider that about a half million go to Canyonlands, and 2.5 million see Glen Canyon each year, and you've got an underutilized facility at your disposal.

There are 13 sites at the park's campground. They're nothing fancy, but they each provide the necessary accommodations—a table and a place to set up your tent. There's no water in the camp, but water and modern restrooms are available at the visitor's center less than a quarter of a mile away on a footpath that leaves directly from the campground. You will have garbage and recycling service, so if Natural Bridges is one stop on your Tour-de-Southern-Utah road trip, you can unload your empties here with a clean conscience. The park is actually very eco-friendly; it runs on solar power collected from an array that's on display for public viewing.

Site 5 is probably the belle of the ball in the campground, with 1 through 4 and 6 taking their place at her side. Avoid sites 7 through 9; they're a bit crammed in there and a little more open to the scorching sun. Although the campground is open all year, summers can sizzle this far south. Come during fall, spring, or even winter to avoid a nasty sunburn and a sweat-soaked sleepless night.

All sites are first come, first served. If you didn't arrive in time to be served, there is overflow camping

> *Kachina Bridge could fit the Great Sphinx or the Mayflower's top mast under her span.*

RATINGS

Beauty: ✿ ✿ ✿
Privacy: ✿ ✿ ✿
Spaciousness: ✿ ✿ ✿ ✿
Quiet: ✿ ✿ ✿
Security: ✿ ✿ ✿ ✿
Cleanliness: ✿ ✿ ✿ ✿

ADDRESS:	Natural Bridges National Monument HC-60 Box 1 Lake Powell, UT 84533
OPERATED BY:	National Park Service
INFORMATION:	(435) 692-1234; www.nps.gov/nabr
OPEN:	Year-round
SITES:	11
EACH SITE HAS:	Picnic table, barbecue stand, tent pad
ASSIGNMENT:	First come, first served
REGISTRATION:	Self-register on-site
FACILITIES:	Vault toilets, garbage, recycling
PARKING:	At site only
FEE:	$10 per night, $5 extra vehicle
ELEVATION:	7,379 feet
RESTRICTIONS:	1 vehicle, 3 tents, 8 people per site

back at the junction of UT 95 and UT 261, as well as dispersed camping along Deer Flats and Bear's Ears roads. Camping along UT 275 is prohibited. Nearly all of the land surrounding the park is federal Bureau of Land Management (BLM) land, with the exception of the Abajo Mountain Range to the northeast, which is administered by the Forest Service and holds its very own allure.

There are three significant natural bridges in the park: Sipaupu at 220 feet tall, Owachomo at 210 feet, and Kachina, measuring in at 106 feet. To give you some perspective, the park distributes a flyer comparing the heights of these bridges to other known landmarks. The Statue of Liberty, from the top of the torch to the bottom of her feet, would fit underneath both Sipaupu and Owachomo bridges, with about 60 feet to spare. The Taj Mahal would also fit beneath these two bridges. Kachina Bridge could fit the Great Sphinx or the Mayflower's top mast under her span, with 20 or 30 feet of breathing room. Only Rainbow Bridge, located to the southeast near Lake Powell, can best these bridges. The U.S. Capitol building could just squeeze underneath that 290-foot behemoth.

That all sounds dandy on paper, but you just won't grasp how big they are until you see them in person. Luckily, the park is set up for you to do just that. The park's road, Bridge View Drive, turns into a one-way loop just past the campground. Rangers advise you to set aside an hour or so to make the 9-mile circle; that leaves you with time to stop at each bridge's view area to snap a few pictures.

To get the full effect of these expansive natural formations created by the scouring erosion of moving water over vast lengths of time, get out of the car and walk to the base of each bridge. The longest hike is 1.5 miles round-trip, so you won't have to dedicate a major portion of your day to each one. They are moderately strenuous hikes, however. Each one will require you to hike over uneven steps, and both Kachina and Sipaupu employ the use of handrails and ladders.

Foot trails also connect the bridges for more adventurous hikers, or you may opt to explore Horse Collar Ruin. This ancestral Puebloan site is believed to

MAP

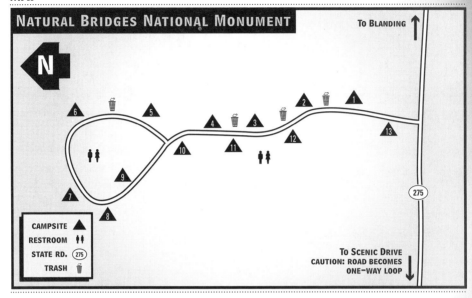

NATURAL BRIDGES NATIONAL MONUMENT

To Blanding

N

275

CAMPSITE
RESTROOM
STATE RD. 275
TRASH

To Scenic Drive
CAUTION: ROAD BECOMES
ONE-WAY LOOP

have been abandoned about 700 years ago, but is in a remarkable state of preservation as a real-life lesson in ancient architecture. Take the advice of park officials and pack at least one gallon of water per person, per day. Disturbing the ruins or climbing on the bridges is, of course, prohibited.

Too many tourists pass by Natural Bridges "on their way to … " or "coming back from … " Don't be one of them. Plan on taking a detour and spending the night at Natural Bridges National Monument to marvel at some of the best natural formations in the world.

GETTING THERE

From Blanding, drive 30 miles west on UT 95, then take UT 275 5 miles to the campground, approximately 1 mile past the park gates.

GPS COORDINATES

UTM Zone: 12
Easting: 589728
Northing: 4162894
Latitude: N 37.60877
Longitude: W 109.98340

33
CEDAR CANYON CAMPGROUND

> *Cedar Canyon is probably best enjoyed from the comfort of a camp chair while sitting around the fire.*

CEDAR **C**ANYON **C**AMPGROUND is the epitome of off-the-highway family camping. Just 13 miles from nearby Cedar City, it's a special little place by the side of the road that allows young and old campers alike to reconnect with nature.

Set amidst spruce, fir, and aspen trees, some of the campsites here get plenty of shade and block out views of the traffic on nearby UT 14. Crow Creek lies between the campsites and the highway as well. Its delightful little song also mutes out the sounds of cars as well as other campers.

Crow Creek is not a fishable stream, but anglers need not despair. Only a few miles farther up the highway there are many different fishing opportunities. At only 11 miles away, Navajo Lake is a fun day trip. There are campgrounds closer to this skinny lake, but they tend to be a bit more raucous than Cedar Canyon. Navajo Lake has the ability to produce quality rainbow, brook, and splake trout (a hybrid of brook and lake trout); but has been hampered in recent years by drought. With a few good water years, this oft-overlooked fishing hole could churn out some big brutes.

Fishing isn't really the main draw at Cedar Canyon; it's the good old-fashioned camping that brings people up UT 14. The sites are spurred along a paved road. About a quarter of the 19 sites are to the left of the entrance road, the rest to the right. The sites could be better masked from each other, but they provide plenty of space to spread your gear, stretch out, and relax.

There are sites to accommodate most family or group sizes here. Just make sure you pay attention when picking your site. Sites 5, 9, 12, 15, and 18 are doubles, and 19 is a triple. If you want to make a reservation ahead of time, only sites 4, 6, 7, 17, and the triple site 19 are available for reservations. All the others are on a first-come, first-served basis.

RATINGS

Beauty: ☆ ☆ ☆ ☆
Privacy: ☆ ☆ ☆
Spaciousness: ☆ ☆ ☆ ☆
Quiet: ☆ ☆ ☆
Security: ☆ ☆ ☆
Cleanliness: ☆ ☆ ☆ ☆

The campsites here are worn in, but not worn down. Actually, the campground is tidy and well maintained. The drinking water is fresh—piped in from a nearby spring—and the toilets are shipshape. There are enough open areas here that kids or anxious adults can spread out and explore. With its location, pleated up against the hill behind it, and a healthy mix of open air and wooded space, Cedar Canyon could host a killer game of steal the flag.

While staying at Cedar Canyon, take the opportunity to visit nearby Cedar Breaks National Monument. Go east on UT 14 about 5 miles and turn left at the junction with UT 148. The monument entrance is 4 miles north on UT 148.

Cedar Breaks is simply stunning. Here you'll see a gargantuan amphitheater carved from the eroded Pink Cliffs of the Claron formation. At its high point, the rim of the massive valley sits at 10,000 feet above sea level, but the canyon plunges 2,000 feet before your eyes. See the dramatic contrast between the pinkish layered canyon walls and the dark green Englemann spruce and subalpine firs that dot the rim and tumbling landscape before you.

Visit Cedar Breaks in early July and you'll also see great colors of blossoming wildflowers in the meadows. Among the most common are bright yellow sunflowers and potentilla, blue lupine and bluebells, and purple larkspur, although the time and focus of your visit will dictate what colors you see.

Cedar Canyon Campground is near the Virgin River Rim Trail—a 32.5-mile trail that parallels UT 14 and is becoming quite popular with mountain bikers. Doing the whole trail by bike in one day is probably too ambitious, but sections can be done as an out-and-back. Start from either the Woods Ranch Recreation Area a few miles below the campground, or the Strawberry Point trailhead located 9 miles up Forest Service Road 60 (Strawberry Road), about 20 miles farther up UT 14. This trail is one of Dixie National Forest's best-kept secrets for exceptional canyon hiking and photography.

While it is surrounded by all kinds of adventure, Cedar Canyon is probably best enjoyed from the comfort of a camp chair while sitting around the fire,

KEY INFORMATION

ADDRESS:	Dixie National Forest Cedar City Ranger District 1789 North Wedgewood Lane Cedar City, UT 84720
OPERATED BY:	Dixie National Forest
INFORMATION:	www.fs.fed.us/r4/dixie
OPEN:	Late May–October (depending on weather)
SITES:	19
EACH SITE HAS:	Picnic table, fire ring
ASSIGNMENT:	By reservation or first come, first served if available
REGISTRATION:	Reserve online at www.reserveamerica.com or call (877) 444-6777; self-register on-site if available
FACILITIES:	Vault toilets, drinking water, garbage service
PARKING:	At site only
FEE:	$12 single sites, $20 double sites, $25 triple site; extra vehicles 50% of site cost each
ELEVATION:	7,940 feet
RESTRICTIONS:	*Pets:* Leashed

MAP

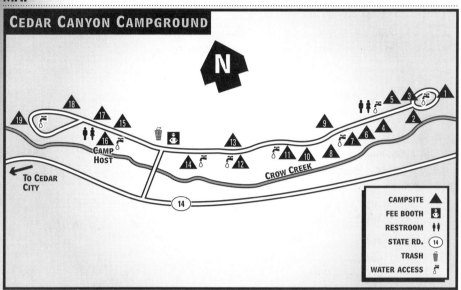

CEDAR CANYON CAMPGROUND

CAMPSITE	▲
FEE BOOTH	🏷
RESTROOM	♙♟
STATE RD.	⑭
TRASH	🗑
WATER ACCESS	🚰

GETTING THERE

From Cedar City, drive 13 miles east on UT 14 to the campground.

marshmallow roaster in hand. The soothing river and crisp mountain air can lull even the most hard-core thrill seeker into a roasted marshmallow–induced sleep.

GPS COORDINATES

UTM Zone: 12
Easting: 331875
Northing: 4162187
Latitude: N 37.59141
Longitude: W 112.90431

34
OAK GROVE CAMPGROUND

HAVE YOU EVER TAKEN A LONG DRIVE up a hot and dusty road and feared what you'd find at the end? Isn't it great when the drive pays off and you find a spectacular new place you never even dreamed could exist? While it's a shame to take the suspense out of your drive to Oak Grove, I have to share that this hidden little campground is an unexpected happy ending to what first appeared an unpromising journey.

The road to Oak Grove will give you a firsthand lesson about the effects of elevation on plant life. After leaving Leeds and the tiny town of Silver Reef, the landscape is tan and drab with only a few freckles of dark green juniper and scrubby sage. As the dusty dirt road winds farther up Leeds Creek, however, wildflowers appear—sporadically at first, then in profusion—and the journey begins to show promise. Flowering cacti line the road, and the fold of earth around the creek is a verdant vein that shimmies from side to side with each bend in the riverbed. As you near the campground, the oak trees appear. Then, as if on cue, the great ponderosa pine trees come into sight, forming a wall that surrounds the campground and protects the Pine Valley Mountain Wilderness. Welcome to Oak Grove Campground.

As the crow flies, you're now less than 4 miles from the Pine Valley Recreation Complex. This Forest Service land holds three campgrounds, a picnic area, and the small Pine Valley Reservoir. The problem is, you've got a 3,500-foot vertical cliff between you and that recreation complex. You'll soon come to realize that the cliff isn't really a problem at all—rather a blessed buffer between you and the many OHVs, trailers, and constant drone of activity up on top. Oak Grove moves at a slower pace than the other Pine Valley campgrounds.

> *Oak Grove moves at a slower pace than the other Pine Valley campgrounds.*

RATINGS

Beauty: ✿ ✿ ✿ ✿ ✿
Privacy: ✿ ✿ ✿ ✿
Spaciousness: ✿ ✿ ✿ ✿
Quiet: ✿ ✿ ✿ ✿
Security: ✿ ✿ ✿ ✿ ✿
Cleanliness: ✿ ✿ ✿ ✿ ✿

ADDRESS:	Dixie National Forest
	Pine Valley Ranger District
	196 East Tabernacle, Suite 40
	St. George, UT 84770
OPERATED BY:	Dixie National Forest
INFORMATION:	www.fs.fed.us/r4/dixie
OPEN:	Mid-May–October (depending on weather)
SITES:	8
EACH SITE HAS:	Picnic table, fire pit, barbecue stand
ASSIGNMENT:	First come, first served; no reservations
REGISTRATION:	Self-register on-site
FACILITIES:	Vault toilets, drinking water
PARKING:	At site only; group parking for day use
FEE:	$5 per night
ELEVATION:	6,380 feet
RESTRICTIONS:	*Pets:* Leashed

If you decide that you do want to go check out the Pine Valley Recreation Complex, you'll have to work to get there on foot. Take the Oak Grove Trail from the trailhead in camp and you'll work your way up a steep incline, then around the side of the cliffs before mounting a straight ascent on the Browns Point Trail. You'll have views of Zion National Park and even northern Arizona mountains from this 6-mile trail, but every snapshot will be paid for by your burning legs and heavy breathing.

With more than 50,000 acres under the federal wilderness designation, you've got plenty of hikes to choose from. The Summit Trail follows the backbone of Pine Valley mountain for 18 miles, or you can bag Washington County's highest peak, Signal Peak, at 10,365 feet.

The campsites at Oak Grove provide enough space and privacy to keep you happy, except perhaps sites 4 through 6. Double site 5 is planted on the side of the road where the line between road, parking lot, and campsite becomes blurred. Still, the campground is quiet enough that even these sites are OK. Set up camp in site number 1 to stay away from the other sites. You'll have to hoof it to the parking area by site 2 for water, but privacy is worth the sacrifice. Site 8 is also removed from the rest, and also has a mysterious wooden gazebo nearby. Exactly why a wooden gazebo sits at the edge of the campground is never explained, but it is a nice bonus feature, especially if you're camping with somebody you love.

Oak Grove isn't immune from OHVs. Back down the dirt road toward town, OHVs have left their mark and are a popular place for locals to pull back on the throttle. According to Forest Service rules, however, they aren't allowed to be ridden inside the campground boundaries, and above the camp is designated wilderness where they are strictly forbidden.

Fishing opportunities are pretty scant in this neck of the woods. Leeds Creek holds a small population of native Bonneville cutthroats, which were actually transplanted from the other side of the mountain. Tributaries to Leeds Creek like Pig Creek, Horse Creek, and Spirit Creek are also accessible by foot and have some

MAP

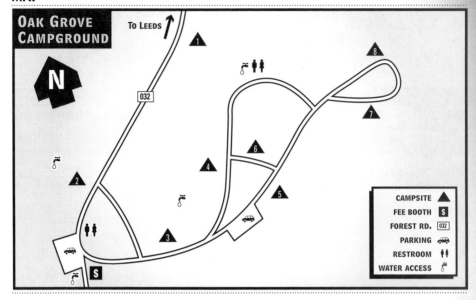

OAK GROVE CAMPGROUND

To Leeds

N

032

CAMPSITE	▲
FEE BOOTH	S
FOREST RD.	032
PARKING	🚗
RESTROOM	🚻
WATER ACCESS	🚰

of the small trout. Practice catch and release in these waters to help the growing population of Bonnies get established.

Oak Grove is on the doorstep of Utah's second-largest wilderness area, yet your chances of being alone here are extremely high. Pine Valley Mountain beckons you to explore its unsung trails and rugged beauty. Discover a new favorite camping spot, drink from a refreshingly cold spring, and take advantage of all that Oak Grove has to offer.

GETTING THERE

From Interstate 15, take the Leeds exit and go northwest on Silver Reef Road. Pass all the homes and continue on the pavement-turned-dirt Forest Service Road 32 for 9 miles to the campground.

GPS COORDINATES

UTM Zone: 12
Easting: 282784
Northing: 4132911
Latitude: 37.31749
Longitude: W 113.45132

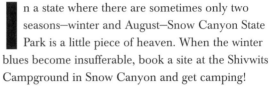

> *When the winter blues become insufferable, book a site at the Shivwits Campground.*

I n a state where there are sometimes only two seasons—winter and August—Snow Canyon State Park is a little piece of heaven. When the winter blues become insufferable, book a site at the Shivwits Campground in Snow Canyon and get camping!

Less than 15 miles (as the crow flies) from the Arizona border, Snow Canyon encompasses just more than 5,700 acres of dramatic rolling canyons, which can vary in color from very deep, dark reds, to hues of tan, gold, and even white. Crowning large areas of this colored Navajo sandstone are large twisted veins of black lava rock formed by three separate episodes of ancient volcanic activity.

Ironically, Snow Canyon rarely sees any snow, so it's an ideal place to go when other campgrounds are snowed in or just too cold. Temperatures can dip at night during the colder months, but it's the daytime weather that attracts the crowds. A good sleeping bag and a knit beanie will probably do the trick to get you through the night, although you'll probably want to get up and get moving early. Most campsites are shaded for a long time in the morning due to their location against the large and rounded stone cliffs that serve the campground's backdrop.

Shivwits Campground is more or less a large figure eight pressed up against the side of a sandstone cliff. Turn in from the park's main road and you'll immediately see the park office. Continue to your right for sites 1 through 19, or left to the quieter sites 20 through 29.

Sites 1 through 14 are set aside for RV use only. These sites resemble a drive-through more than a campsite, but suit RVers who are looking for a place to park and be hooked up. These RV sites remain isolated from the individual tent sites located on both ends of the figure eight and quickly blend in with other structures near the campground entrance.

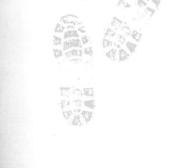

RATINGS

Beauty: ✿ ✿ ✿ ✿
Privacy: ✿ ✿ ✿
Spaciousness: ✿ ✿ ✿
Quiet: ✿ ✿ ✿
Security: ✿ ✿ ✿
Cleanliness: ✿ ✿ ✿ ✿ ✿

The tent sites here are liberally spaced, and, wherever possible, inserted among the trees and high shrubbery to allow for the most privacy. In particular, sites 17, 20 through 22, and 26 through 29 will keep you sheltered from the views of others and enhance your outdoors experience. Showers and modern restrooms are available, so you won't completely escape the modern world. But just being outdoors in the middle of January or February will unquestionably feel good regardless.

Much of the park's focus is directed to the different rocks and its unique geology, but each campsite has been prepared with a soft sandy spot to set your tent. Although you may want to build a roaring fire to keep warm, check with officials about current fire restrictions. Drought and fears of devastating fire have led to the prohibition of fires from June through the middle of September.

The same volcanic activity that deposited black and gray rock flows also left the park with lava tubes and caves that beg to be explored. The Butterfly Trail is a moderate 2-mile trail that leads to West Canyon Overlook and some of the park's famous lava tubes. Exploring any lava tubes or caves can be risky business, so use good judgment and always err on the side of caution.

For a slightly less intimidating hike, take the Pioneer Names Trail. When pioneers came through Snow Canyon in the late 1800s, some stopped to write their names in axle grease. Their names remain on the sandstone face, some dating back to 1883. The half-mile trail is relatively level and takes you right to the pioneer autographs.

Most trails are open to hikers, bikers, and horsemen alike. Rock climbing, however, has become a large part of the recreation in the park. Park officials have asked that visitors not climb the rocks behind the campground, but instead seek approved places to scale the sandstone. If you're new to climbing, there is a local outfitter that conducts technical climbing classes in the park. Check with a park ranger for details about climbing classes and current climbing regulations.

Don't think that the cold months are the only time to come to Snow Canyon. If you want to explore and

KEY INFORMATION

ADDRESS:	Snow Canyon State Park 1002 Snow Canyon Drive Ivins, UT 84738
OPERATED BY:	Utah State Parks and Recreation
INFORMATION:	www.stateparks .utah.gov
OPEN:	Year-round
SITES:	29
EACH SITE HAS:	Picnic table, barbecue stand
ASSIGNMENT:	Two-thirds by reservation; one-third first come, first served
REGISTRATION:	Reserve online at www.reserve america.com or call (800) 322-3770; self-register on-site
FACILITIES:	Flush toilets, drinking water, garbage service, showers
PARKING:	At site only
FEE:	$15–$18
ELEVATION:	3,400 feet
RESTRICTIONS:	*Fires:* Prohibited June 1–September 15 *Other:* Tents on pads only

MAP

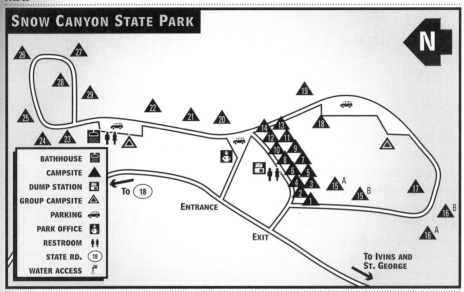

SNOW CANYON STATE PARK

BATHHOUSE
CAMPSITE
DUMP STATION
GROUP CAMPSITE
PARKING
PARK OFFICE
RESTROOM
STATE RD.
WATER ACCESS

To (18)

ENTRANCE

EXIT

TO IVINS AND
ST. GEORGE

GETTING THERE

From Interstate 15 take the
Bluff Street/UT 18 north exit
to St. George. Drive northwest on UT 18 approxi-
mately 12 miles to the park
entrance.

avoid the biggest crowds, July and August are sure to
meet your needs. Temps often reach above 100°F and
only slip to 70°F at night, but you will find a little more
breathing room than you normally would in April or
October.

While your neighbors lock themselves into their
home for another winter evening full of sappy prime-
time programming and stuffy recirculated air, stay at
the Shivwits Campground in Snow Canyon State Park
and camp when you never thought it was possible.

GPS COORDINATES

UTM Zone: 12
Easting: 265638
Northing: 4120665
Latitude: N 37.20305
Longitude: W 113.64078

36
RED CLIFFS CAMPGROUND

IN **1996** AN **IMPRESSIVE COALITION** of federal and state land managers, cities, environmental groups, and local counties realized the need to protect the fragile ecosystem of southwestern Utah, and so united to create the Red Cliffs Desert Reserve. Some 62,000 acres were set aside to protect animals like the desert tortoise—federally listed as "threatened"—and other varieties of wildlife on the state's "sensitive species list" of animals that have become increasingly pressured by rapid population growth and heightened recreational land use.

Today, the land reserve represents a magnificent opportunity for some of the best desert camping and hiking in the state. Start your adventure in the Red Cliffs Desert Reserve by staying at Red Cliffs Campground. It's the ideal place to get hydrated and rest for a day of desert hiking.

Although temperatures on the reserve can soar well above 100°F in the summertime, you'll find some relief at Red Cliffs. Tiny little Quail Creek (sometimes referred to as Harrisburg Creek) trickles down through the campground most days, providing just enough moisture for a thriving population of giant cottonwoods along the banks. These trees and the protective red cliffs of the campground's namesake are enough to take the edge off of insufferable summer heat. The canyon walls also keep the winds down, making the campground a superb place to plan a camping trip when the rest of the state is just too cold. Beware of sudden rainstorms, though, as the creek can rise dramatically with just a few minutes of intense rain, rendering the road back to town impassable.

Scattered under the cottonwoods alongside the campground's main road loop are 11 typical Bureau of Land Management (BLM) campsites, each with a table, fire ring, and barbecue stand. A few of the less-shaded

> *Start your adventure exploring a magnificent desert reserve from Red Cliffs Campground.*

RATINGS

Beauty: ✿ ✿ ✿ ✿ ✿
Privacy: ✿ ✿ ✿ ✿
Spaciousness: ✿ ✿ ✿ ✿
Quiet: ✿ ✿ ✿
Security: ✿ ✿ ✿ ✿
Cleanliness: ✿ ✿ ✿ ✿

ADDRESS:	Bureau of Land Management St. George Field Office 345 East Riverside Drive St. George, UT 84790
OPERATED BY:	Bureau of Land Management
INFORMATION:	www.ut.blm.gov/ stgeorge_fo/sgfored_ cliffs.html
OPEN:	Year-round
SITES:	11
EACH SITE HAS:	Picnic table, fire pit, barbecue stand
ASSIGNMENT:	First come, first served; no reservations
REGISTRATION:	Self-register on-site
FACILITIES:	Vault toilets, drinking water, some shade awnings available
PARKING:	At site only; group parking for day use
FEE:	$8 per night, $2 day use
ELEVATION:	3,120 feet
RESTRICTIONS:	None

sites also have a shade awning over the picnic table. One of the real pluses of this campground is the availability of drinking water. Spigots are generously placed over the grounds ensuring that you never have to walk far to fill your canteen.

Try to snatch up site 10. It's the last site on the loop and sits right near the creek with its own water spigot and plenty of sand to serve as a comfy cushion under your tent. Just be mindful of the rain. Although it didn't appear to show signs of frequent flooding, this site sits close enough to the water that it can't help but be at risk of getting a little damp from time to time. Sites 4 and 5 are on much higher ground, although they're closer to the other sites and offer little protection from the sun.

There are three trails that leave from the campground. The Silver Reef Trail is a short uphill jaunt leading to the overlook of the Silver Reef area where silver was mined in the early 1900s. The half-mile interpretive trail will help you identify the plant species around you, and the Red Cliffs Village Trail takes you to an old Anasazi ruin dating back to 1000 A.D. Each trail is easy to hike even for young children, but each closes at dusk.

For more-adventurous hikes, head into the Red Cliffs Desert Reserve, accessible near the campground on the road back to town. The boundaries are clearly marked and you'll know when you've reached the reserve's edge. "Step-overs" placed at entrances to the reserve are not only physical reminders of the special land designation, but mental reminders of the special hiking, biking, and equestrian regulations. By crossing a step-over, visitors also acknowledge their responsibility to help protect the fragile desert ecology by not interfering with the wildlife. For more information on specific regulations, see the reserve's Web site at **www.redcliffsdesertreserve.com.**

The Red Cliffs Desert Reserve sits at the crossroads of three distinct ecosystems: the Mojave Desert, Great Basin, and Colorado Plateau. That gives the land here an eclectic collection of inhabitants like the desert tortoise, Gila monster, chuckwalla, and sidewinder rattlesnake. Sensitive species alone number 45, some of

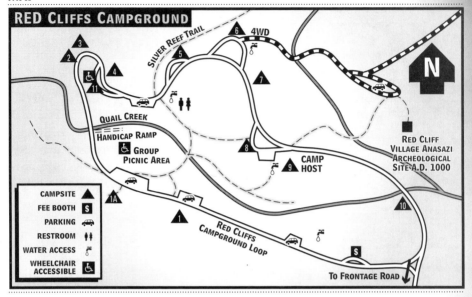

which are only known to exist here in the desert pre-serve. Be mindful of your surroundings, and be espe-cially vigilant to look out for any of the venomous snakes in the area. Most don't bother humans unless provoked, but snakes have little interest in discerning if your provocation came on purpose or by accident.

The flora of Red Cliffs is also a hodgepodge of plant life from three different ecosystems. Look for the healthy population of blackbrush, more commonly found in cooler climates, or one of the species of yucca and cacti that flourish at Red Cliffs. You'll also have a good chance to snap a photo of Utah's official state flower, the sego lily.

Serious hikers will appreciate the convenience of Red Cliffs, families will enjoy the picniclike atmo-sphere of its shady river bottom, and anyone can wel-come the shelter this campground provides during both the hottest and the coldest Utah months.

GETTING THERE

From Interstate 15, take the Leeds exit and go south on the frontage road to the town of Harrisburg. Turn right at the Red Cliffs recreation signs and go west under-neath the freeway and 2 miles to the campground.

GPS COORDINATES

UTM Zone: 12
Easting: 286711
Northing: 4122319
Latitude: N 37.22300
Longitude: W 113.40400

> *Zion is a Hebrew word meaning refuge or sanctuary, and that's exactly what Lava Point is.*

PERCHED HIGH IN THE KOLOB TERRACE section of Zion National Park is the quiet and unassuming Lava Point Campground. Few people venture to this section of the park, and those who do aren't visiting by accident. Lava Point is where serious park visitors, especially hikers, make camp. It's the capital of the *other* Zion National Park.

While countless campers clog the crowded streets near the Zion Canyon Visitor Center, Lava Point remains blissfully unaware. As you make the turnoff on Kolob Road near the town of Virgin, you get the feeling that you know something no one else does. The turn is not well marked, and the road passes through a small residential area before ascending along North Creek.

Climbing along the creek you will enter and exit park boundaries two separate times. It's easy to tell when a boundary has been crossed, as the road changes color; Zion roads are red-hued asphalt, state roads are black. The changing colors beneath you, however, pale in comparison to the changing colors of the environment around you. Your 4,000-foot ascension will take you from scrubby brown and olive bushes through thick, light green trees, around massive gray and tan bulbous rock knobs, and near high-plateau farms. Near the end of the 30-mile road you'll see a bright blue reservoir and find Lava Point Campground.

Zion is a Hebrew word meaning refuge or sanctuary, and that's exactly what Zion's Lava Point is. It's a small, single-loop campground with only six primitive sites and views to knock your socks off. This is an aspen-guarded refuge from the 2.5 million visitors that come to Zion each year.

The campsites here are flat and mostly shaded, with convenient garbage service and adequate space to spread your things. They are set a bit too close together, but the quiet in the surrounding air is contagious, and

RATINGS

Beauty: ✩ ✩ ✩ ✩
Privacy: ✩ ✩ ✩
Spaciousness: ✩ ✩ ✩ ✩
Quiet: ✩ ✩ ✩ ✩ ✩
Security: ✩ ✩ ✩ ✩ ✩
Cleanliness: ✩ ✩ ✩ ✩

most campers can't help but speak in reverent whisper. The loudest noise you're bound to hear on your visit may be the buzzing of the flies and other pesky bugs. Bring plenty of spray or even a head net. At this campground these insects thrive for most of the summer and can quickly drive you mad.

Next to the camp is the Lava Point overlook. Here you'll get gorgeous views of the Horse Pasture Plateau as it fades from pine and white fir to juniper and short shrubs. The views have been enhanced by an aggressive restoration project undertaken to reduce the amount of invasive white fir trees and help reestablish the aspen population. For the next several years it may look like the 45-acre section lost a fight with a chainsaw, but in the long run, park officials hope it will encourage new aspen trees to grow and reduce fire risk caused by overly dense fir forest.

Most visitors to Lava Point come with one hike in mind: the West Rim Trail. This 14-mile (one-way) trail connects Lava Point and the Kolob Terrace section of the Park with the main canyon, passing views of many side canyons like Potato Hollow and the Great West Canyon, and passing through Refrigerator Canyon. This hike is usually done over two days. Trying to complete it in one just means you won't have time to take all the photos you'd like—a serious mistake on this trail.

Make sure you acquire the proper permits before heading out on any hike. Because of the intense pressure this park receives, permits are required for all overnight trips, all the thru-hikes of the Narrows and its tributaries, and several other widely used hikes in the park. The most popular hikes, the Subway and Mystery Canyon, are only given on a lottery basis. The park has set up a Web site for permits at **www.zionpermits .nps.gov.** Take the time to read through it thoroughly when planning a visit and always have a backup plan if you can't get a permit for the area you'd like.

Recreation isn't bound to park-related attractions. Just 3 miles from Lava Point is Kolob Reservoir, a special-regulations fishery that has been producing some impressive cutthroat trout in the past few years. Early morning and pre-dusk fishing seem to be the key here, although with the right fly you could catch your

KEY INFORMATION

ADDRESS:	Zion National Park UT 9 Springdale, UT 84767-1099
OPERATED BY:	National Park Service
INFORMATION:	www.nps.gov/zion
OPEN:	June–October (depending on weather)
SITES:	6
EACH SITE HAS:	Picnic table, fire ring, garbage can
ASSIGNMENT:	First come, first served; no reservation
REGISTRATION:	Self-register on-site
FACILITIES:	Vault toilets, drinking water, garbage service
PARKING:	At site only
FEE:	None (national park entrance fee required)
ELEVATION:	7,870 feet
RESTRICTIONS:	None

MAP

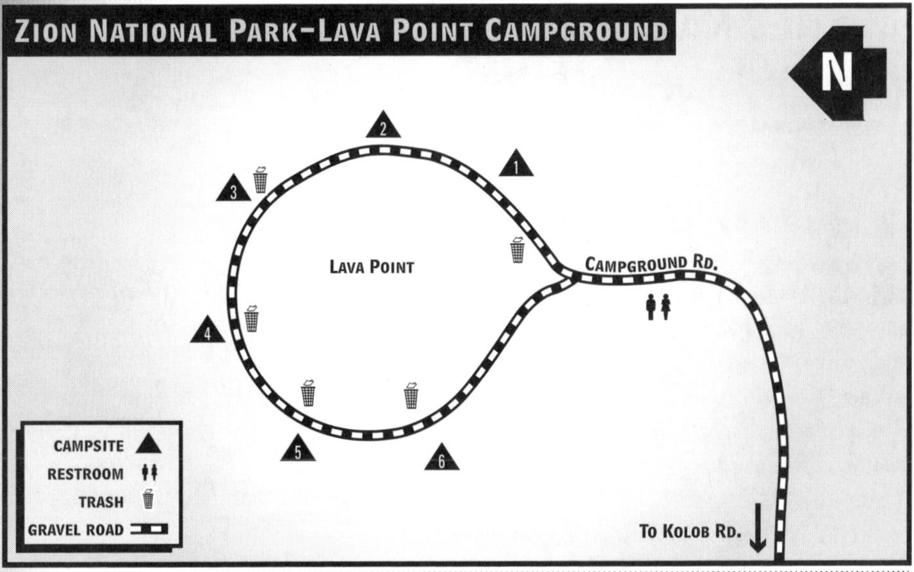
ZION NATIONAL PARK–LAVA POINT CAMPGROUND
N
LAVA POINT
CAMPGROUND RD.
TO KOLOB RD.
1
2
3
4
5
6
CAMPSITE
RESTROOM
TRASH
GRAVEL ROAD

GETTING THERE

Turn off UT 9 in the town of Virgin and go north on Kolob Road for about 25 miles. Just before Blue Springs Reservoir, turn right and follow a short dirt road to the campground.

GPS COORDINATES

UTM Zone: 12
Easting: 320019
Northing: 4139337
Latitude: N 37.38333
Longitude: W 113.03294

limit at practically any hour. Just be sure to take the paved Kolob Road all the way to the end to find Kolob Reservoir. Blue Springs Reservoir near the campground may look alluring, but private cabin owners are quite adamant about keeping it private.

If you're staying at Lava Point for several days, just give in and visit the main canyon area along UT 9. Be aware that in summer the area is accessible by shuttle bus only and can take some time to explore. Crowds aside, hiking through the Virgin River in the main canyon is a fun way to spend an afternoon. Depths range from "sloshy shoes" to "over your head." You'll definitely have to be on your toes.

For a real gut-check, try the Angel's Landing Trail. Acrophobics need not attempt the skinny trail with chain handrails. It takes hikers 1,700 feet up a rugged red knob and leaves them with dizzying, adrenaline-enhanced views.

Zion National Park is the busiest of all Utah national parks, but you'd never know it from staying at Lava Point. Here the cacophony of cars and tourists is replaced by the quaking of aspen leaves and the quiet of the *other* Zion National Park.

38
ARCHES NATIONAL PARK-HITTLE BOTTOM CAMPGROUND

HITTLE BOTTOM CAMPGROUND sits only 6 miles from the eastern edge of Arches National Park, but to get there you'll pass the turnoff to the park on US 191, turn up UT 128, and then drive 30 miles to reach it. As you make your way up the Colorado River on sinuous UT 128, enjoy the spectacular sights, from the verdant riparian riverway to the soaring sandstone spires. The drive is definitely worth it.

Hittle Bottom is a true hidden gem—far enough away from the bustle of Moab and Arches to give you a peaceful camping experience, yet close enough that you can access any of the area's main attractions with only a short commute.

Arches National Park is an obvious day-trip destination if you're based at Hittle Bottom. Arches is relatively small at just under 75,000 acres, but it is unlike any other place on earth in its concentration of naturally occurring arches. At last count, it held more than 900 of them, with more likely to be discovered. These airy openings in otherwise solid stone walls excite the imagination of park visitors and set the perfect backdrop frame for anyone who wants to take a photo.

Delicate Arch is the flagship of Arches, and in more recent years, the poster child for Utah tourism. The likeness of Delicate Arch can be seen on local business logos, bumper stickers, and even on the new Utah license plates. This 33-foot-long, 45-foot-high arch sits on the rim of a large and steep-sided bowl. Ribbons of orange, tan, and buff run horizontally across the legs of the arch, adding details and highlights to the structure that keep you examining the formation over and over again. It's easy to see why many consider this one feature the single most-photographed item in Utah.

To reach Delicate Arch, enter the park from the turnoff just north of Moab on US 191 and take the

> *Enjoy the spectacular sights, from the verdant riparian riverway to the soaring sandstone spires.*

RATINGS

Beauty: ✿ ✿ ✿ ✿ ✿
Privacy: ✿ ✿ ✿ ✿
Spaciousness: ✿ ✿ ✿ ✿ ✿
Quiet: ✿ ✿ ✿ ✿
Security: ✿ ✿ ✿ ✿
Cleanliness: ✿ ✿ ✿ ✿

KEY INFORMATION

ADDRESS: Hittle Bottom Campground Bureau of Land Management Moab Field Office 82 East Dogwood Moab, UT 84532

OPERATED BY: Bureau of Land Management Moab Field Office

INFORMATION: www.blm.gov/utah/moab

OPEN: Year-round

SITES: 9

EACH SITE HAS: Picnic table, metal fire ring

ASSIGNMENT: First come, first served; no reservation

REGISTRATION: Self-register on-site

FACILITIES: Vault toilets, paved boat launch

PARKING: 2 vehicles per site; grouped parking sites

FEE: $10 per night

ELEVATION: 4,021 feet

RESTRICTION: *Pets:* Leashed *Fires:* In rings only *Other:* 2 vehicles, 4 tents, 10 people per site; no wood collecting

paved road 11 miles to the junction for Wolfe Ranch and Delicate Arch. Turn right on this road and continue about a mile to the Wolfe Ranch parking area. Park and hike the 1.5 miles over steep slickrock to Delicate Arch for an up-close and personal view. Bring plenty of water and avoid going in the heat of the day as there's scarcely any shade. Better yet, go in the evening and see the arch at sunset.

If you can't make the 3-mile round-trip, just continue on the paved road past Wolfe Ranch for less than a mile to the Delicate Arch Viewpoint parking area. Here you can find more information at an interpretive display and enjoy the view of the arch from a distance. Or opt for a 1.5-mile round-trip hike to see the arch from a different vantage point.

Fiery Furnace is another popular hike in the park. This area showcases the "fins" of sandstone canyons—long rock peninsulas that tower above the canyon floor and drop off dramatically on each side. Park rangers offer guided walks of Fiery Furnace and recommend that no one enter on their own. Many hikers have become lost in the labyrinth of narrow trails. Those who do enter on their own must obtain a permit from park officials. To access Fiery Furnace, go back to the main park road and continue about 2.5 miles deeper into the park to the turnoff for Fiery Furnace. Talk to park officials at the visitor's center located at the park entrance to find out when guided tours of Fiery Furnace depart each day.

With landmark names like "Park Avenue," "Balanced Rock," "Devil's Garden," and "Dark Angel," you could spend days pursuing new adventures in Arches. Just be mindful of the park rules. Recent actions of attention-hungry individuals have caused the park service to tighten regulations; most notably they have reemphasized that visitors are strictly prohibited from climbing on any named arch inside the park. Obey the rules and take home photographs instead of fines—they make better souvenirs.

At the end of the day when most park visitors are jamming into the park's Devil's Garden Campground, you can make your way back to Hittle Bottom and rest quietly for the night. With only 10 sites, you won't have

MAP

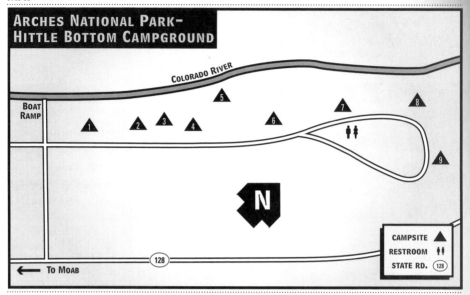

ARCHES NATIONAL PARK– HITTLE BOTTOM CAMPGROUND

COLORADO RIVER

BOAT RAMP

1 2 3 4 5 6 7 8 9

N

CAMPSITE ▲
RESTROOM ♦♦
STATE RD. (128)

128

← TO MOAB

big crowds at night. You'll enjoy special seclusion by avoiding sites 2 through 4, which are right next to each other. Site 5 is tucked back beneath a tall cottonwood and surrounded by tamarisks, and site 9 is located all by itself on the end of the campground loop.

If you don't want all the commotion of a national park, you can lounge around camp and enjoy the view of Fisher Towers, or put in your raft or kayak on the site's paved boat ramp. If you do enter the water, make sure you know what's downstream. The Colorado River may look calm, but its swift-moving waters can be dangerous, especially during spring runoff.

GETTING THERE

Take Interstate 70 exit 182 (US 191 South) 29 miles to Moab. Turn left on UT 128 and drive 23 miles east to the campground.

GPS COORDINATES

UTM Zone:12
Easting: 645621
Northing: 4291383
Latitude: N 38.75915
Longitude: W 109.32402

> *This high-mountain campground is the perfect place to make your home base.*

PINE LAKE IS A DAY-TRIPPER'S DREAM. It's located within a few hours' radius of two national parks, three state parks, and two national monuments, so time is the only restraint on how much exploring you can do. This high-mountain campground is the perfect place to make your home base and maximize your time in what is arguably Utah's most sensational outdoors corridor.

Aptly named for its location among spruce and towering ponderosa pine trees, Pine Lake is a cool and out-of-the-way spot in an otherwise hot and busy region of southern Utah. Most of the spots here are shaded and have good access to drinking water—a rarity among the region's more out-of-the-way camp-grounds. At more than 8,100 feet in elevation, Pine Lake's nights will be brisk but a welcome change to warmer days. The only downside is that the camp-ground doesn't typically open until Memorial Day or later, depending on the weather.

Pine Lake Campground has an upper and lower loop that piggyback one on top of the other. Sites 3 through 14 and 28 through 33 are located on the lower loop, 15 through 27 on the upper. About half of the individual sites here can be reserved ahead of time (3 through 5, 14 through 17, 26 through 30, and 32), as well as the group areas. The campsites fill up on the weekends, so make your reservations ahead of time to ensure you've got a place to stay. If not, dispersed camping is allowed beyond the lake, but sites are harder to find and more frequently buzzed by OHVs along the Great Western Trail.

If you're staying during the week, try getting any site in the upper loop (except 22, which is right on the road). These cannot be reserved but are farthest away from the host, the lake, and other campers. If you'd rather get close to the water, try the lower loop,

RATINGS

Beauty: ✿ ✿ ✿ ✿
Privacy: ✿ ✿ ✿
Spaciousness: ✿ ✿ ✿ ✿
Quiet: ✿ ✿ ✿ ✿
Security: ✿ ✿ ✿ ✿
Cleanliness: ✿ ✿ ✿ ✿

although if you're reserving a site, 32 is the closest reserved site you can get.

One of the best features of the campground is its proximity to Pine Lake. The shores of the lake are only a few minutes away—close enough to visit when you'd like, but far enough away that campers with little ones won't have to keep looking over their shoulder.

This pretty little lake is a great place to launch a canoe and get out on the open water. At 77 acres in surface area, you've got plenty of space to paddle. Since powerboats of any kind are prohibited, arm power rules the lake. Take along a fishing pole and try for one of the lake's resident rainbow or cutthroat trout. They can be a bit finicky, but can usually be coaxed into playing tug-of-war when they get hungry at sunup and sundown.

Check current fishing regulations before wetting your line. Pine Lake has been the focus of some habitat restoration work in years past, and special regulations were placed to protect spawning trout, including the closure of the river that flows into the lake.

With each new day started at Pine Lake Campground you have the best of southern Utah recreation at your fingertips. Most Pine Lake campers spend at least one day at Bryce Canyon National Park. The entrance to the park is just 17 miles away, back down UT 22. The National Park Service recently created a shuttle service for Bryce Canyon, which means you'll drive just half an hour to the gates, park your car, and then take a bus into the park.

Bryce Canyon is truly a treat for the imagination. The exceptional geology of this area has earned it the honor of being one of Utah's most stellar places to snap a photo. Large spires defy gravity as they claw their way upward to the sky. The limestone rock has been so eroded that countless canyons, windows, and fins have been created here in the Paunsaugunt Plateau.

Other day trips might include Kodachrome Basin, Escalante, or Anasazi State Parks to the east along UT 12. Grand Staircase-Escalante National Monument and Capitol Reef National Park are also found to the east on UT 12.

KEY INFORMATION

ADDRESS:	Dixie National Forest Escalante Ranger District 755 West Main Street Escalante, UT 84726-0246
OPERATED BY:	Dixie National Forest
INFORMATION:	www.fs.fed.us/r4/dixie
OPEN:	Late May–October (depending on weather)
SITES:	33
EACH SITE HAS:	Picnic table, fire ring
ASSIGNMENT:	About 50% reserved; 50% first come, first served
REGISTRATION:	Reserve online at www.reserveamerica.com or call (877) 444-6777; individual sites self-register on-site
FACILITIES:	Vault toilets, drinking water, primitive boat launch
PARKING:	At site only
FEE:	$9 per night, $4 additional vehicle fee, $2 day use
ELEVATION:	8,150 feet
RESTRICTIONS:	*Pets:* Leashed

MAP

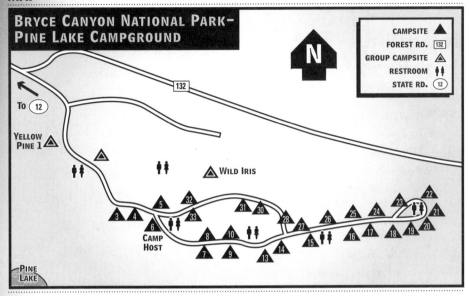

BRYCE CANYON NATIONAL PARK– PINE LAKE CAMPGROUND

CAMPSITE ▲
FOREST RD. 132
GROUP CAMPSITE ⚠
RESTROOM ♂♀
STATE RD. 12

To 12

YELLOW PINE 1

WILD IRIS

CAMP HOST

PINE LAKE

GETTING THERE

From Tropic, drive 7.5 miles west on UT 12. At the junction with Bryce Canyon National Park, turn right and travel approximately 10 miles north on UT 22. Turn right at the signed marker and drive 7 miles on a dirt road to the campground.

GPS COORDINATES

UTM Zone: 12
Easting: 416100
Northing: 4178011
Latitude: N 37.74555
Longitude: W 111.95232

Consider driving UT 12 itself as a worthwhile day trip. This stretch of highway is often considered to be the most beautiful road in the United States as it wanders over narrow fins and narrowly carved rock face.

To the west, Red Canyon and Cedar Breaks National Monument are doable day trips. Both are postcard-worthy destinations that will have your photo finger clicking. Although a campground does exist at Red Canyon, you'll be glad you're up at Pine Lake when you see (and hear) the crowds that pass through the area immediately surrounding that area.

Plan your next family reunion at Pine Lake Campground and you'll be the family hero. There are five reservation group sites that cater entirely to the needs of family groups, with large open areas away from the waterfront and nearby water spigots and restrooms for convenience. Rather than sit around and listen all week long to stories about Aunt Margie's latest medical procedure, you'll be able to escape to a different adventure each day, or just head to the lake. The fresh air and comforting scenery should help you shake out of your head the images of Aunt Margie in a hospital gown.

40
CAPITOL REEF NATIONAL PARK–FRUITA CAMPGROUND

FRUITA **CAMPGROUND** in Capitol Reef National Park offers a one-of-a-kind camping experience. Where else can you view the marvels of a singular and gorgeous national park *and* wander through orchards eating ripe fruit to your belly's content?

As its name suggests, Fruita Campground sits among fruit–22 orchards spread over more than 60 acres that were first planted by Mormon pioneers as they settled the nearby community of Fruita in 1880. The National Park Service now maintains the approximately 2,700 trees as a Rural Historic Landscape, growing cherries, apricots, peaches, pears, apples, plums, mulberries, almonds, and walnuts.

The campground itself is in the heart of all the orchards and consists of three loops tucked between the Fremont River and road. Loops A and B sit right near the river and its footpath, while Loop C is separated from the river by the amphitheater.

Each campsite is a spur off of the paved loop road and sites are positioned one next to the other. There is a graveled parking space next to the lawn where you'll set up your tent. True, you'll feel like you're at a park more than a campground, with the large shade trees and ubiquitous green grass, but giving up stillness and solitude are a fair trade for the experience of staying here.

Stay at the campground and you can take advantage of the park's official invitation, as found in one of the park's brochures: "You are welcome to stroll in any unlocked orchard and you may consume as much ripe fruit as you want while in the orchards." As much ripe fruit as you want! Bring on the cherries! Bring on the apricots! Bring on the Pepto Bismol!

If you'd like to take home some genuine Capitol Reef fruit for friends and neighbors, there are self pick-and-pay stations for any fruit you take home. Some visitors plan their trips around the harvest time of their

> *Phenomenal scenery, fabulous hiking, and free fruit combine for a truly fantastic camping experience.*

RATINGS

Beauty: ✪ ✪ ✪ ✪
Privacy: ✪ ✪
Spaciousness: ✪ ✪
Quiet: ✪ ✪
Security: ✪ ✪ ✪
Cleanliness: ✪ ✪ ✪ ✪

ADDRESS: Capitol Reef
National Park
HC 70, Box 15
Torrey, UT 84775

OPERATED BY: National Park
Service

INFORMATION: www.nps.gov/care

OPEN: Year-round

SITES: 71

EACH SITE HAS: Picnic table,
barbecue stand

ASSIGNMENT: First come, first
served

REGISTRATION: Self-register on-site;
group site reserved
in advance—call
(435) 425-3791

FACILITIES: Flush toilets,
drinking water,
visitor center

PARKING: At campsite;
overflow parking
available

FEE: $10 per night

ELEVATION: 5,400 feet

RESTRICTIONS: *Pets:* Leashed
Fires: Prohibited
Other: 8 people per
site

favorite fruit. Although weather can change availability, the schedule below shows the approximate flower and harvest dates of different fruits. For current fruit conditions, call the park's fruit hotline at (435) 425-3791.

	FLOWERING	HARVEST
Cherries	3/31–4/19	6/11–7/7
Apricots	2/27–3/20 early	6/27–7/22 early
	3/7–4/13 regular	6/28–7/18 regular
Peaches	3/26–4/23	8/4–9/6
Pears	3/31–5/3	8/7–9/8
Apples	4/10–5/6	9/4–10/17

Each of the 71 sites available here is on a first-come, first-served basis. In summer, the camp fills up quickly so plan to show up early if you want a site. On the weekends it's sure to fill, so even showing up on Friday morning is risky. Do yourself a favor: Take that extra day off work and get into Fruita by Thursday morning. You'll avoid the risk of finding the campground full and you'll have an extra-long weekend to enjoy the area.

Capitol Reef National Park is most famous for the 100-mile wrinkle in the Earth's surface that it sits on, known as Waterpocket Fold. This "kink" in the Earth's crust, created by the same force that lifted the Colorado Plateau, is home to brightly colored cliffs, rock spires, domes, arches, and monoliths that defy the imagination.

Hikers enjoy a multitude of opportunities and some of the finest desert hiking available in the state. Cathedral Valley in the northern part of the park is accessible only by dirt road—from the west over the Thousand Lake Mountains (see chapter 46), or from the east on rocky roads that ford various rivers. Massive monoliths define this region of Capitol Reef. Muley Twist Canyon, a popular attraction in the south of the park, is a challenging desert hike that will have you discovering exciting arches and new views around every turn.

Camping in the backcountry is allowed, but a free permit must first be acquired from park officials. Be prepared for rough conditions on any hike or backcountry adventure. Water is scarce in many parts of the park, so bring plenty of your own.

MAP

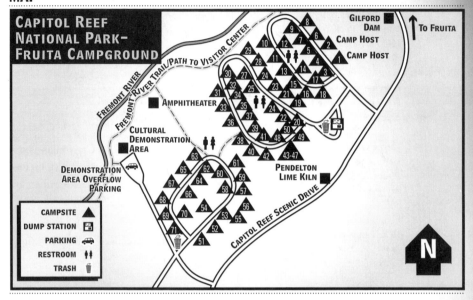

CAPITOL REEF NATIONAL PARK– FRUITA CAMPGROUND

FREMONT RIVER TRAIL/PATH TO VISITOR CENTER

FREMONT RIVER

GILFORD DAM
CAMP HOST
CAMP HOST

↑ TO FRUITA

AMPHITHEATER

CULTURAL DEMONSTRATION AREA

DEMONSTRATION AREA OVERFLOW PARKING

PENDELTON LIME KILN

CAPITOL REEF SCENIC DRIVE

CAMPSITE ▲
DUMP STATION
PARKING
RESTROOM
TRASH

N

If you'd rather not take on the trails of Capitol Reef, there's plenty to do around Fruita Campground. Take the 25-mile round-trip scenic drive to view Waterpocket Fold from the comfort of your own car. This two-hour outing leaves from the campground and puts you into some inspiring landscape. Be sure to get the printed drive guide from the visitor center before you go.

Near the campground, some of the original structures built by early settlers have been restored and are open to view. Tour the old Fruita Schoolhouse, blacksmith shop, Gifford Homestead, and Ripple Rock Nature Center. Many cultural presentations, children's activities, and handmade sales items are offered each day. Check with the visitor center for a detailed schedule.

The diversity of Utah's camping opportunities is never illustrated better than at Fruita in Capitol Reef National Park, where phenomenal scenery, fabulous hiking, and free fruit combine for a truly fantastic camping experience.

GETTING THERE

From Torrey, drive 11 miles east on UT 24 to the entrance of Capitol Reef. Turn right and go 1.5 miles south past the visitor center to the campground.

GPS COORDINATES

UTM Zone: 12
Easting: 478259
Northing: 4237232
Latitude: N 38.28289
Longitude: W 111.24859

41
CANYONLANDS NATIONAL PARK– HAMBURGER ROCK CAMPGROUND

If this giant sandstone rock is a hamburger, you'll be sleeping with the pickles and mayo!

HAMBURGER ROCK CAMPGROUND is certainly one of the most unique campgrounds in Utah. Just minutes from the official Canyonlands National Park boundary is a squatty, circular stone formation that, with the right tilt of your head—and on an empty stomach—bares a striking resemblance to a hamburger with all the fixin's.

This burger's not just for looks; you can dive right into one of the Bureau of Land Management's (BLM) seven campsites that are tucked into the nooks and crannies of the burger's perimeter. These tiny alcoves provide shelter from the sun and wind, and keep you separated from other campers.

In colder months, you may want to set up camp in either site 2 or site 3. You'll have the warm sunshine in camp for most of the day. The tradeoff is privacy, which dissipates in these two less-protected sites. Site 1 is definitely the most unique site in the campground. If this giant sandstone rock is a hamburger, you'll be sleeping with the pickles and mayo! It's as though a small wedge has been nibbled away and site 1 tucks into the rounded rock formation. On the back side of the campground, sites 4 and 5 are also structured similarly, though to a lesser degree.

Amenities are lean here; only a pit toilet on the east side of the campground and convenient road access set it apart from primitive dispersed camping in the region. However, the toilet is tidy and quite a luxury where the vegetation is sparse. And come on, how cool is it to say you've camped in a hamburger?

Normally a bulgy little burger would look out of place, but Hamburger Rock fits in well here in the Indian Creek area. Just a mile and a half farther down Lockhart Road in the BLM's all-but-abandoned Indian Creek Campground, the scenery really gets wild. There are flat, chocoloate-chunk cliff walls,

RATINGS

Beauty: ✰ ✰ ✰ ✰
Privacy: ✰ ✰ ✰ ✰
Spaciousness: ✰ ✰ ✰
Quiet: ✰ ✰ ✰
Security: ✰ ✰ ✰ ✰
Cleanliness: ✰ ✰ ✰ ✰ ✰

funky toadstool rock stands, and far-off mesas that form a perfect backdrop.

On my last visit (when I missed Hamburger Rock in the dark and rain), my wife and I stayed dispersed-style at a little C-shaped alcove now aptly nicknamed Fortune Cookie campsite. While we had made the journey in the dark of night, we awoke the next morning to a cloudless sky and our first vision of the area by daylight. Breathtaking! Vibrant red and orange hues contrasted against the profoundly deep blue sky, and we saw hundreds of tiny pools of water that filled the pockmarked sandstone surfaces surrounding us. This is the scenery in the Indian Creek area.

Plan on staying at Hamburger Rock for a while; there's plenty to explore. Most Hamburger Rockers do it by OHV, but you'll be better rewarded on foot. UT 211 hosts a bevy of trailheads, both marked and unmarked. Follow UT 211 a few more miles and you'll enter the Needles District of Canyonlands National Park where there are day hikes of all shapes and sizes, and some of Utah's best backpacking possibilities. Your best bet is to find a good guidebook specific to the Canyonlands area and whittle down your choices. Also, the Canyonlands Web site has great overview maps available in PDF format for downloading. Be vigilant in verifying park regulations regarding backcountry hiking and camping. Permits are required and in some cases must be reserved well in advance.

The drive to Hamburger Rock will test your tendency to stop and smell the roses. The sweetest rose along this journey is Newspaper Rock, which sits just off of UT 211 about 12.5 miles from the junction with US 163. Newspaper Rock is a smooth and dark sandstone rock face peppered with petroglyphs dating back perhaps some 2,000 years. They are not exclusive to one culture; Anasazi, Fremont, Navajo, and more modern Anglo symbols are all represented in this hodgepodge of ancient writings. Whether it was an ancient newspaper or bulletin board, or held a more sacred role, no one knows for sure. Take a few minutes to gaze at the hundreds of petroglyphs on your way to the campground to make your own judgment.

KEY INFORMATION

ADDRESS:	Bureau of Land Management Monticello Field Office 435 North Main Monticello, UT 84535
OPERATED BY:	Bureau of Land Management
INFORMATION:	(435) 587-1500; www.blm.gov/utah /monticello/ camping.htm
OPEN:	Year-round
SITES:	7
EACH SITE HAS:	Picnic table, fire ring
ASSIGNMENT:	First come, first served
REGISTRATION:	Self-register on-site
FACILITIES:	Vault toilets
PARKING:	At campsite only
FEE:	$6 per night
ELEVATION:	4,866 feet
RESTRICTIONS:	2 vehicles per site

MAP

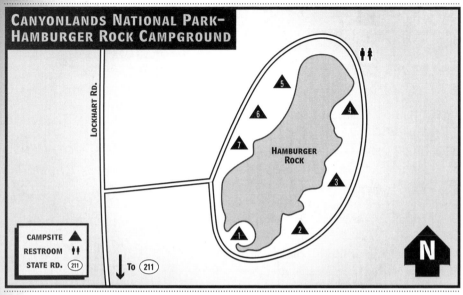

**CANYONLANDS NATIONAL PARK–
HAMBURGER ROCK CAMPGROUND**

LOCKHART RD.

5

6

4

7

HAMBURGER
ROCK

3

CAMPSITE ▲
RESTROOM ♦♦
STATE RD. (211)

1

2

To (211)

N

GETTING THERE

From Monticello, go 14.5 miles north on US 163 and turn left on UT 211 (Canyonlands Access). Go approximately 29 miles west, turn right on Lockhart Road, and go 1.5 miles north to the campground.

Lockhart Road is easy to miss. It's an unassuming little turnoff marked only by a small informational kiosk a few hundred feet down the dirt road directly off of UT 211 on the right-hand side. The last time I was in the area I did manage to find the turnoff in the dark, although I passed right by the campground. Allow a few extra minutes just in case, pay attention, and you'll be just fine. For the GPS crowd, the turnoff is at N 38.17552 W 109.66630.

GPS COORDINATES

UTM Zone: 12
Easting: 616443
Northing: 4227959
Latitude: N 38.19205
Longitude: W 109.67028

42
HORSETHIEF
CAMPGROUND

STEALING HORSES IN THE **19**TH CENTURY was hard work. Thieves pilfered them from Moab ranchers in the La Sal Mountains and drove them west across the dry and dusty trail toward the Henry Mountains Range. Horsethief Campground marks the area where they turned the stolen goods southwest to cross the distant Green River on their way to Robber's Roost.

Today, this site holds 56 campsites on three loops named for notable Western horse breeds/colors: Buckskin, Cayuse, and Appaloosa. As you enter the campsite from the road, Buckskin and Cayuse loops are on your left. For privacy, your best bets are the more distanced sites 44 through 50 on the Cayuse Loop, although privacy is a relative term in the pinyon-juniper forests of southeastern Utah. Scrubby juniper and sage do little to shield you from your neighbor or provide shade from the sun. Decide when you want your shade—morning or evening—then pick your site accordingly.

Campsites on the south side of the Appaloosa loop boast the best views of the gentle slope and the small ridge that's located about a half mile from the camp. If you want a better view of the distant Henry Mountains, take the short, well-marked hike out to the ridge. It's less than a mile, and the trailhead is on the Appaloosa loop between sites 13 and 14.

Although the wild and wide-open public lands near this campground beg for exploring, Horsethief Campgrond's true value lies in its proximity to some of the area's more established destinations. Visit Dead Horse Point State Park, just 10 miles away. Here you'll be reminded that it's not heights you should be afraid of, but rather depths. You'll enjoy awesome views from the edge of a cliff that plunges 2,000 feet to the Colorado River below. According to one legend, horses came to this point and were so thirsty they jumped off

> *Horsethief Campground's true value lies in its proximity to some of the area's more established destinations.*

RATINGS

Beauty: ✰ ✰ ✰
Privacy: ✰ ✰
Spaciousness: ✰ ✰ ✰
Quiet: ✰ ✰ ✰ ✰
Security: ✰ ✰ ✰ ✰ ✰
Cleanliness: ✰ ✰ ✰ ✰ ✰

ADDRESS: Horsethief Campground Bureau of Land Management Moab Field Office 82 East Dogwood Moab, UT 84532

OPERATED BY: Bureau of Land Management Moab Field Office

INFORMATION: www.blm.gov/ utah/moab

OPEN: Year-round

SITES: 56

EACH SITE HAS: Picnic table, metal fire ring

ASSIGNMENT: First come, first served; no reservations

REGISTRATION: Self-registration on-site

FACILITIES: Vault toilets, garbage service, gravel road

PARKING: 2 vehicles per site, at campsites only

FEE: $10 per night

ELEVATION: 5,842 feet

RESTRICTION: *Pets:* Leashed *Fires:* In rings only *Other:* 2 vehicles, 4 tents, 10 people per site; no firewood collecting

the high plateau to reach the water below, hence the park's grisly name.

Views are especially breathtaking at sunrise and sunset when the light creeps up and down the jagged canyon walls, igniting them in brilliant hues of orange and red before leaving them in a glorious silhouette against the night sky. Check the information board at the visitor's center where the staff updates the time for sunrise and sunset daily.

Although the Dead Horse Point does have its own campground, it's a bit cramped and crowded and can get a little loud. On my visit it was full, while Horsethief had only 2 of its 56 sites occupied.

Horsethief Campground also puts you a mere 7 miles from the boundaries of Canyonlands National Park. The park is divided into three districts: Needles, Maze, and Island in the Sky; the latter is accessible from Horsethief by continuing down UT 313 for another 7 miles. Make sure you go straight past the turnoff to Dead Horse Point.

The Island in the Sky District of Canyonlands is known for its stunning vistas that showcase layer upon layer of colorful canyons. Most are accessed from the convenience of your car on large turnouts from the district's main paved road. Bring your camera to snap some shots of Shafer Canyon, Green River, and Grand View Point Overlooks. Although photos can't do justice to the buttes, bluffs, and beautiful canyons you'll see, your friends will still have fits of jealousy when you show them your snapshots.

Leave the paved road and you'll be rewarded with exceptional hiking opportunities and more solitude than you'd expect in a national park. For an easy but more popular hike, follow the signs to the Mesa Arch trail. This short loop hike gives you a closer look at a small arch without leaving you out of breath.

Canyonlands receives surprisingly light hiking pressure, probably due to the rugged nature of many of its hikes, especially in the Maze District. Here the trailheads are even difficult to reach via four-wheel drive vehicles, but experienced hikers relish the challenge of conquering more remote backcountry. The opportunities are too many to name, so do your

MAP

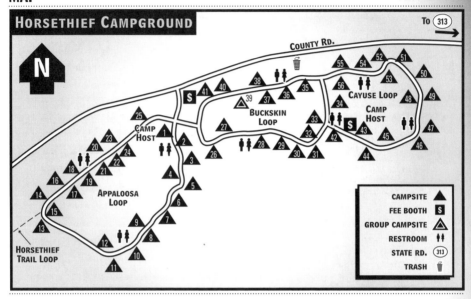

HORSETHIEF CAMPGROUND

To (313) →

COUNTY RD.

BUCKSKIN LOOP

CAYUSE LOOP

CAMP HOST

CAMP HOST

APPALOOSA LOOP

HORSETHIEF TRAIL LOOP

CAMPSITE	▲
FEE BOOTH	S
GROUP CAMPSITE	△
RESTROOM	♀♂
STATE RD.	(313)
TRASH	🗑

research before you set out. Bear in mind that water can be scarce in the park and dangerous conditions exist. Talk with park officials about your plans and make sure you obtain a backcountry permit for any backpacking you'll be doing. Reservations for permits aren't necessary, but are strongly recommended to avoid disappointment. Call the national park reservation office at (801) 259-4351 for more information.

Horsethief Campground is a great place to lay in your tent and make last-minute plans for the adventure you're about to have or dream about the one you just did. Stay during any season but the scorching summer and you'll have a comfortable and calm place to hang your hat. Listen closely and you may even hear the footsteps of old outlaws with their herd of stolen horses.

GETTING THERE

Take Interstate 70 exit 182 (US 191 South) 21 miles to UT 313. Take UT 313 12 miles to the campground.

GPS COORDINATES

UTM Zone:12
Easting:603277
Northing:4271302
Latitude: N 38.58419
Longitude: W 109.81424

> *However you enjoy Lonesome Beaver, you'll be one of the few who has.*

LONESOME BEAVER IS CERTAINLY AN ODDITY, but not in a bad way. Its location deep in southern Utah, coupled with the fact that it's a Bureau of Land Management (BLM) campground, would lead you to believe it's a dusty-desert locale full of sage, pinion pine, and plenty of hot temperatures. Au contraire. This small, secluded campground in the Henry Mountains is literally an oasis in southern Utah.

At more than 8,000 feet in elevation, Lonesome Beaver is placed square in the middle of a forest—truly an out-of-character place to find a BLM campground. A small river runs alongside the campsites here. Although fishless, it still provides a pleasant song for campers and plenty of inspiration for your imagination to create its own "Legend of the Lonesome Beaver" tale. No one seems to know the real story.

There are five sites here surrounded by tall trees you wouldn't typically associate with the Lake Powell area of Utah—among them Douglas fir, spruce, ponderosa pine, and aspen. A bevy of smaller plant life also dots the landscape to add to the surprise of the Henries.

The fauna surrounding the area is perhaps what makes Lonesome Beaver so atypical. The Henry Mountains are the only place in the lower 48 states to find a free-roaming herd of American bison that are still hunted. The state issues a few dozen permits each year, so chances of getting a shot are slim. For better odds, talk to the Henry Mountains field office about where you might catch a peek at the herd and have a chance to shoot a few photos.

Mountain lions, mule deer, rabbits, and numerous bird species also call this unique place their home. When I arrived at the campground, it was full of wild turkeys. I counted more than 30, although it could have easily been more. (Have *you* ever tried counting a

RATINGS

Beauty: ✩ ✩ ✩ ✩
Privacy: ✩ ✩ ✩
Spaciousness: ✩ ✩ ✩
Quiet: ✩ ✩ ✩ ✩
Security: ✩ ✩ ✩ ✩
Cleanliness: ✩ ✩ ✩ ✩ ✩

rafter of turkeys while they're excited about the human thing chasing them with a camera? Not easy.)

The Henry Mountains seem to rise up out of the desert and beckon the adventurous traveler to come to its fingered canyons. Geologists delight in the unique formation of the steep mountainside. It's believed that molten lava pushed its way upward but could not break the thick layer of earth crust. Instead, the crust only bulged without rupturing to create "laccoliths"— the five prominent peaks of the Henries. Over time, erosion has exposed the now-hardened diorite core of the mountain. Visitors can explore different areas of the mountain to see these formations and the transitions to more typical geology in the surrounding area.

One of the best ways to enjoy the Henry Mountains is to take the alternate route to the campground along Bull Mountain Road and over Wickiup Pass. Catch Bull Mountain Road off of UT 95, about 20 miles south of Hanksville. You'll climb steadily right up the mountainside, getting a chance to peer east over Glen Canyon National Recreation Area and driving through a massive burn area to see the power of fire up close and personal.

Bull Mountain Road was actually in better condition than Sawmill Basin Road on my visit, though heavy rains, winter damage, and maintenance schedules could affect that. Bring a high-clearance vehicle just to be sure.

Although not everyone signs in at the campground kiosk, it's noteworthy that I was just the fifth person to sign the camp register all year, and I made my visit *after* Labor Day when there was already snow in the peaks. You've got a good chance at some alone time here. Even the BLM doesn't make too many trips to the campground, so be extra vigilant in maintaining and cleaning up your campsite.

Below the campground is the Dandelion Flats day-use area. It appears this picnic and play area is frequented more often than the campground, and would make an excellent day trip for anyone looking for a brief respite from the heat of nearby Lake Powell on their extended camping trip.

KEY INFORMATION

ADDRESS:	Bureau of Land Management Henry Mountains Field Station 380 South 100 West Hanksville, UT 84734
OPERATED BY:	Bureau of Land Management
INFORMATION:	(435) 542-3461; www.publiclands .org
OPEN:	May–October
SITES:	5
EACH SITE HAS:	Picnic table, barbecue stand, fire pit
ASSIGNMENT:	First come, first served
REGISTRATION:	Self-register on-site
FACILITIES:	Vault toilets, drinking water
PARKING:	At campsite only
FEE:	$4 per night
ELEVATION:	8,230 feet
RESTRICTIONS:	*Fires:* In rings only *Other:* 14-day stay limit

MAP

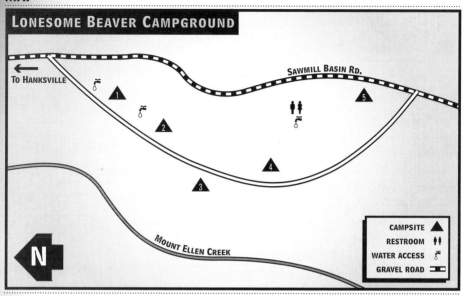

LONESOME BEAVER CAMPGROUND

To Hanksville

SAWMILL BASIN RD.

MOUNT ELLEN CREEK

CAMPSITE	▲
RESTROOM	♂♀
WATER ACCESS	🚰
GRAVEL ROAD	▭

N

GETTING THERE

From Hanksville, go 34 miles south on the graveled-then-dirt Sawmill Basin Road (100 West) to the campground.

There are a few trails in the area for hiking enthusiasts. Visit Bull Mountain Pass and take the 4-mile trail to Mt. Ellen. At 11,600 feet, you get spectacular views of the surrounding desert. Or, leave from Dandelion Flats and go 4 miles around a Mt. Ellen ridge.

However you enjoy Lonesome Beaver, you'll be one of the few who has. With such a singular personality and unique geology, this is one campground that will call out to you until you come for a visit.

GPS COORDINATES

UTM Zone: 12
Easting: 519450
Northing: 4218001
Latitude: N 38.10962
Longitude: W 110.77814

WITH DOLLAR SIGNS IN HIS EYES, a hopeful Al Starr came to the southern tip of the Henry Mountain in the 1880s in search of mining fortunes. Instead, Starr was met with a cruel reminder of how unforgiving the untamed west can be. His mine never produced any ore, and he was forced to close down the operation when drought and locoweed (a toxic plant that wreaks havoc on an animal's nervous system) killed most of his horses.

Today conditions are much more hospitable at Starr Springs, although there are still reminders, besides the campground's name, of Starr's misfortune. Just before arriving at camp you'll see the remnants of a small structure on the left-hand side of the road. A sign there recounts this woeful tale of a once-hopeful miner. The structure was to be the base of his operations, though Starr was defeated by the desert before his buildings could be completed.

Starr Springs Campground is arranged in a single loop of 12 individual sites numbered counterclockwise along the road. Sites 1 through 5 are surrounded by relatively flat land, while sites 6 through 8 back up into a gentle downhill slope populated with thick brush. Sites 9 through 12 return to flat space, but 10 and 11 offer less shade than their counterparts. Still, site 10 is handsome and spacious enough to merit consideration. It's got quick access to water and restroom facilities. Site 5 shares these characteristics and is situated on the inside of the loop.

There's a handy little day-use area found just below the campground on the drive in, with several picnic tables and massive cottonwood trees for shade. The main campground is shaded by the resident oak trees, which do a good job of blocking out the intense heat in this part of the state.

You'll need to call ahead to the Bureau of Land

> *Sneak down to Glen Canyon NRA during the day for some of its overlooked hikes.*

RATINGS

Beauty: ☆ ☆ ☆
Privacy: ☆ ☆ ☆ ☆
Spaciousness: ☆ ☆ ☆
Quiet: ☆ ☆ ☆ ☆
Security: ☆ ☆ ☆ ☆
Cleanliness: ☆ ☆ ☆ ☆

ADDRESS: Bureau of Land
Management
Henry Mountains
Field Station
380 South 100 West
Hanksville, UT
84734

OPERATED BY: Bureau of Land
Management

INFORMATION: (435) 542-3461;
www.publiclands
.org

OPEN: April–November

SITES: 12

EACH SITE HAS: Picnic table,
barbecue stand,
fire ring

ASSIGNMENT: First come, first
served

REGISTRATION: Self-register on-site

FACILITIES: Vault toilets, water

PARKING: At campsite only

FEE: $4 per night

ELEVATION: 6,100 feet

RESTRICTIONS: *Fires:* In rings only
Other: 14-day stay
limit

Management (BLM) to check the status of the drinking water at Starr Springs. The campground is piped for water and has provided service for many years, but it's evident there has been some recent maintenance, perhaps due to problems in the system. The BLM has posted a note at the campground kiosk informing visitors that the water has been shut off and they are uncertain when water service might return.

The small Panorama Knoll Nature Trail begins just north of the campground and gives the curious just a taste of what the Henry Mountains offer by showcasing some of the natural wonders and offering a glimpse at the soaring peak of Mount Hillers. To summit the peak, go back down to the main road and continue to wrap around the hillside toward Stanton Pass. From there, it's pretty much a straight shot up the side of the mountain. The hike will compensate you for your efforts with killer views of Capitol Reef National Park's Waterpocket Fold, a 100-mile-long fold in the crust of the earth.

Keep your eyes peeled for the free-roaming bison herd of the Henry Mountains area, but don't be disappointed if they don't make an appearance; instead, focus on the variety of birds in the region, including a slew of different jays, flycatchers, and vireos.

There's no denying that Lake Powell reigns as the region's most popular attraction. The reservoir, encompassed in the larger Glen Canyon Recreation Area, draws around two and a half million visitors each year. There are two ways to do Powell: the loud way or the quiet way. Both have their merits, but if you stay at Starr Springs you're probably more interested in the quiet way. Sneak down to Glen Canyon NRA during the day for some of its overlooked hikes and side canyon adventures. The park's Web site lists many of the day hikes by region, as well as a few of the park's most popular long hikes. Depending on which area you explore, you could be the only human being for miles. After a day of tranquil hiking, pass by the crowds in the closer campgrounds on your way back to the cooler and more comfortable campground you left that morning.

The loud way—by powerboat, houseboat, or in one of the campgrounds right on the camp's shore—is really a riot. Most Powell devotees do it this way and

MAP

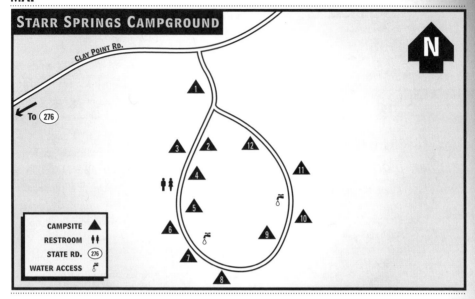

STARR SPRINGS CAMPGROUND

CLAY POINT RD.

To 276

N

CAMPSITE ▲
RESTROOM ♀♂
STATE RD. 276
WATER ACCESS

still manage to fit in a bit of quiet time in one of the fingerlike side canyons the reservoir is famous for. If you're the kind of person who wants to be right in the middle of the action, you'll probably be happier at one of the campgrounds closer to the water.

When most people think of the Henry Mountains, Lake Powell, or Glen Canyon National Recreation Area, they don't think of Starr Springs Campground. Use that to your advantage for an unorthodox tent trip to Utah's summer recreation headquarters.

GETTING THERE

From Bullfrog, go 22 miles northeast on UT 276 to the marked campground turnoff. Continue almost 4 miles on a graded dirt road to the campground.

GPS COORDINATES

UTM Zone: 12
Easting: 529628
Northing: 4189135
Latitude: N 37.84918
Longitude: W 110.66323

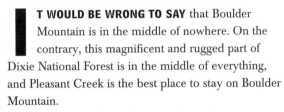

> *Pleasant Creek is the best place to stay on Boulder Mountain.*

IT WOULD BE WRONG TO SAY that Boulder Mountain is in the middle of nowhere. On the contrary, this magnificent and rugged part of Dixie National Forest is in the middle of everything, and Pleasant Creek is the best place to stay on Boulder Mountain.

A quick calculation by a popular online mapping service shows the drive time to the town of Torrey at 3 hours and 44 minutes from the biggest cities of Salt Lake and Washington Counties, the most populated counties of northern and southern Utah, respectively. That means that most Utahns could leave work on a Friday afternoon and be sitting in a camp chair listening to the bubbling waters of Pleasant Creek as it passes by their tent just as the summer sun goes down. Campers from farther away may have to ditch the last hour of work, but that's what Friday afternoons are all about … right?

Pleasant Creek is actually split between two separate campgrounds—upper and lower. The upper is spread around an open loop with each site's parking plot spurred from the main circle. There are 12 first-come, first-served sites surrounded by tall pines reached by crossing Pleasant Creek. Site 4 is ADA accessible, and garbage service is provided throughout.

At the lower campground, things are a bit more intimate. There are only five sites here and they back into Pleasant Creek as it turns away from the highway on its way to delivering water into Lower Bowns Reservoir. The campsites fit snugly together around a shorter loop and are each allotted a bit less space than are the upper sites.

You probably won't encounter any RVs at the lower site. A sign at the entrance advises against them. According to the site host, most RVs actually fly by Pleasant Creek in favor of other nearby campgrounds

RATINGS

Beauty: ✿ ✿ ✿ ✿ ✿
Privacy: ✿ ✿ ✿
Spaciousness: ✿ ✿ ✿ ✿
Quiet: ✿ ✿ ✿
Security: ✿ ✿ ✿
Cleanliness: ✿ ✿ ✿ ✿

like Singletree or Lower Bowns, which are bigger and more accommodating to RV needs. If Pleasant Creek happens to be full, try Oak Creek Campground as a backup, just over a mile south on UT 12. It too caters to tent campers.

It's hard to get locals to talk about "The Boulder." They're fiercely protective of the high-mountain retreat. Perhaps that's why it's rarely visited by anyone but locals and coincidental passersby. Try to pry a favorite fishing hole out of a Boulder Mountain regular and you'd think you were asking for their private bank account number. They're tight-lipped for a reason; some of the biggest brook trout in the state swim in the dozens of lakes on the mountain. The state record brookie, a 7-pound, 8-ounce beast, was caught here in 1978, and the record still stands today. You may just have to buy a topographical map and start exploring all the blue dots. Don't overlook the thin blue lines, though. In addition to holding some great brook and cutthroat trout, the rivers here will lead you to some picture-perfect places, where the elements of a model forest—blue skies, clear water, towering trees—all come together before your eyes.

If you're feeling adventurous, take a drive to the Aquarious Plateau, or "Boulder Top," as it's more commonly known. Be forewarned, however, that the Boulders are appropriately named. What can look like an innocent dirt road to begin with quickly turns into a gnarled, menacing 4x4 experience. These roads are unrepentant in their desire to eat your truck and leave you stranded. High-clearance four-wheel drive vehicles are absolutely required on all off-road excursions.

To reach the Boulder Top, you'll either have to drive to the town of Bicknell and take Posey Lake Road and Forest Service Road 178 south, or drive all the way back down to Escalante and follow the signs north on Forest Service Road 153 to Posey Lake Campground. These roads are typically closed until the middle of June because of snow, so call the Forest Service ahead of time to check conditions. If you've braved the rough roads, you'll find enough hiking and fishing on the Aquarious Plateau to keep you coming back for years.

Stay near camp at Pleasant Creek and you'll still

KEY INFORMATION

ADDRESS:	Fishlake National Forest Fremont River Ranger District 138 East Main P.O. Box 90 Teasdale, UT 84773-0090
OPERATED BY:	AuDi Campground Services
INFORMATION:	www.fs.fed.us/r4/ fishlake/recreation
OPEN:	Mid-May– mid-October, weather permitting
SITES:	17
EACH SITE HAS:	Picnic table
ASSIGNMENT:	First come, first served
REGISTRATION:	Self-register on-site at lower campground
FACILITIES:	Vault toilets, drinking water
PARKING:	At campsite only
FEE:	$9 per night, $4.50 each additional vehicle
ELEVATION:	8,750 feet
RESTRICTIONS:	*Pets:* Leashed *Other:* 14-day stay limit

MAP

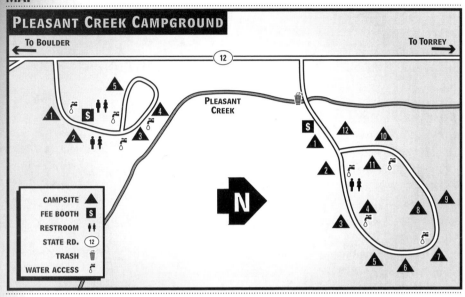

PLEASANT CREEK CAMPGROUND

To BOULDER ←   → To TORREY

12

PLEASANT CREEK

N

CAMPSITE ▲
FEE BOOTH **S**
RESTROOM †††
STATE RD. ⑫
TRASH 🗑
WATER ACCESS ᵟ

GETTING THERE

From Torrey, drive 1 mile east on UT 24. Turn right on UT 12 and go 22 miles south to the campground.

GPS COORDINATES

UTM Zone: 12
Easting: 470499
Northing: 4217044
Latitude: N 38.10072
Longitude: W 111.33647

have plenty of places to drown a worm on a hook. Lower Bowns Reservoir, just a jog from Pleasant Creek Campground, is stocked with always-willing rainbow trout, and many brook trout find their way in from the surrounding tributaries. Within a few minutes' drive, you can access the trail to Oak Creek Reservoir and the nearby Round, Scout, and Long lakes. Farther south still on UT 12 is the trail to Deer Creek Lake and Green, Moosman, and Steep Creek Lakes. There are too many lakes to name, too many trails to detail. Trial and error never sounds so fun as it does here on Boulder Mountain.

It's easy to get into a camping rut—going to the same campgrounds month after month, year after year. There's a simple antidote for same-site syndrome: Pack up the gear and point your car toward Boulder Mountain. It's closer than you think.

46
ELKHORN CAMPGROUND

NO ONE VISITS ELKHORN BY ACCIDENT.
The dirt road to the campground is accessed from a seldom-used stretch of highway and winds continually as it climbs 9 intimidating miles through the trees and passes by deep blue ponds characteristic of the rarely discussed Thousand Lake Mountain. It's remote and it's isolated. In other words, it's almost perfect.

Elkhorn campground is the only established campground on Thousand Lake. The campsites here sit at almost 10,000 feet in altitude in a needle-shaped configuration. Surprisingly, water is available at this campground from several spigots in the camp, and the restrooms appear to have recently been redone to accommodate campers with disabilities.

The only thing that would make Elkhorn better would be spreading the sites out a little farther from each other. Still, being so high above and far away from civilization, you can hardly complain. Bring along your favorite novel—or sit at camp writing your own—and the only distraction you might have would be the overwhelming beauty of the forest around you. The campers and hunters who frequent the mountain also have a quiet respect for one another, so security isn't a big concern. Keep clear of the main road and OHVs won't be a bother, either.

Sites 5 through 7 serve up the best privacy at Elkhorn. They're sheltered from each other by big shady pines. If you've booked the group area (a steal at only $25), you can expect to be out in the open as it's met on its front side by a large meadow and the road to the nearby ranger field station.

Solitude is the main attraction at Elkhorn, and Thousand Lake Mountain offers it in spades. Pick any trail or dirt road and follow it to your explorer heart's content. The only traffic you're bound to see involves

> *Solitude is the main attraction at Elkhorn, and Thousand Lake Mountain offers it in spades.*

RATINGS

Beauty: ✰ ✰ ✰ ✰ ✰
Privacy: ✰ ✰ ✰
Spaciousness: ✰ ✰ ✰
Quiet: ✰ ✰ ✰ ✰
Security: ✰ ✰ ✰ ✰ ✰
Cleanliness: ✰ ✰ ✰ ✰

ADDRESS:	Fishlake National Forest Loa Ranger District 138 South Main Street Loa, UT 84747
OPERATED BY:	Fishlake National Forest
INFORMATION:	www.fs.fed.us/r4/ fishlake/recreation
OPEN:	Memorial Day–Labor Day
SITES:	7 individual, 1 group
EACH SITE HAS:	Picnic table, fire ring
ASSIGNMENT:	First come, first served; group site by reservation
REGISTRATION:	Self-register on-site; group site reserved online at www .reserveusa.com or call (877) 444-6777
FACILITIES:	Vault toilets, drinking water
PARKING:	At campsite only
FEE:	None for individual sites, $25 minimum for group site
ELEVATION:	9,820 feet
RESTRICTIONS:	*Fires:* In rings only

people taking the scenic route over the mountain to Capitol Reef National Park's secluded Cathedral Valley. You'll have passed that turnoff on your way into Elkhorn, so unless you head back down the way you came, you can avoid this group completely.

Consider visiting Cathedral Valley while you're here, though. This awesome part of the national park is accessed on Forest Service Road 22 and boasts some mammoth-size monoliths made of Entrada sandstone that resemble every bit the impressive facades of the world's most ornate cathedrals. Elkhorn is a great place to stage your stay if you like a cooler place to spend your nights. You'll need a high-clearance four-wheel drive vehicle to visit the lonesome and harsh terrain of the sometimes-sandy, sometimes-muddy Cathedral Valley. If you don't have one, at least pull over to the side of the road at one of the many scenic turnoffs on Thousand Lake Mountain and take a picture.

On my visit in the early summer, I had to chuckle at the reservation notice posted on the group site; it was dated for September of the previous year. Apparently, Labor Day weekend was the last time anyone had been at the group area. On the off chance that you do find Elkhorn booked, there are almost infinite places to pull off for dispersed camping—sans the convenience of potties and water.

Near the campground is a small trail leading up the hill to Blue Lake. It's doable by four-wheel drive vehicle, but short enough to be refreshing on foot. It's about a mile-and-a-half hike to Blue, then another 1.5 to Neff Reservoir. You'll also see several small ponds along the way. Bring your fishing pole along and you'll be rewarded by hungry little brook trout. Other stocked lakes in the area include Blind Lake, Deep Creek Lake, Elkhorn Lake, Grass Lake, and Round Lake. Although Thousand Lake Mountain doesn't have as many lakes as Boulder Mountain to the south (in fact, some conjecture that the names of the two were transposed when recorded by early surveyors), there are still plenty of opportunities to test the waters for feisty fishies.

Bring along some bug spray, just to be sure. Nothing will ruin the peace and quiet of this special place

MAP

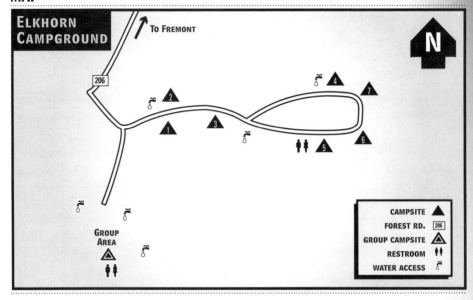

ELKHORN CAMPGROUND

TO FREMONT

N

206

2

4

7

1

3

5

6

CAMPSITE ▲
FOREST RD. 206
GROUP CAMPSITE ⛊
RESTROOM ♟♟
WATER ACCESS ⌁

GROUP AREA

faster than the constant buzz-land-slap routine that mosquitoes evoke. Also be sure to have a good rain jacket and some warmer clothes. You wouldn't think that in a place surrounded by hot and dusty desert you could get that cold, but at 10,000 feet, all bets are off.

Nineteenth-century English poet Christina Rossetti once wrote that, "Silence is more musical than any song." While I don't think she ever visited Thousand Lake Mountain, I am certain that she would appreciate the symphony of silence available at the remote little Elkhorn Campground.

GETTING THERE

From Loa, take UT 72 northeast 10 miles, passing Fremont. Turn right at the signed turnoff and go east 9 miles on a steep and winding dirt road to the campground.

GPS COORDINATES

UTM Zone: 12
Easting: 460123
Northing: 4257364
Latitude: N 38.46370
Longitude: W 111.45709

> *The Abajo Mountains have their own first to claim: first mountains to become snow-free after winter.*

THERE'S A LOT TO BE SAID FOR being first, and the Abajo Mountains (sometimes also called the Blue Mountains) have their own first to claim: first mountains to become snow-free after winter. While the rest of the state languishes under snowpack, Dalton Springs Campground quietly sheds its snow and typically offers some of the first high-mountain experiences for campers and hikers who've been itching with spring fever.

Located just west of the city of Monticello (less than 50 air miles from the border of Arizona) at an altitude of 8,400 feet, this small campground can open as early as the first week of May, according to 35 years of snow-pack data. Compare that to late June or July for the alpine campgrounds in the northern part of the state and you have a perfect destination for a spring when you've just been pining for a campground with pines.

The campground itself is set up as a loop inside of a loop off of Forest Service Road 105. Shaded by pines, oak, and aspen, there are 14 regular campsites and 2 double sites (1 and 14). Sites 4 through 13 are located on an inner loop with numbers 5, 7, 8, and 11 offering pull-through convenience. Stay in site 9, 10, or 12 and you'll be a bit removed from the camp by backing up toward the mountain. Sites 15 and 16 are also nice, though somewhat less private and you'll have to walk farther to get water from 16.

There's plenty to do in the Abajo Mountains. Just up the road past Buckboard Campground (a viable option if Dalton Springs is full) are Monticello and Foy Lakes. Both are quite small but offer fun fishing for planted rainbow trout. Monticello Lake is just off the road. Foy is straight past the fork. The unobstructed views at Foy Lake, which is located at the crest of a hill, are especially noteworthy because of the lake. Look off into the distance and watch the mountains

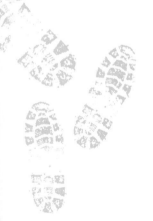

RATINGS

Beauty: ✰ ✰ ✰ ✰
Privacy: ✰ ✰ ✰
Spaciousness: ✰ ✰ ✰
Quiet: ✰ ✰ ✰
Security: ✰ ✰ ✰ ✰
Cleanliness: ✰ ✰ ✰ ✰

tumble down to the valley and turn shades of amber and red.

Drive around to the south side of the mountain toward Nizhoni campground and you'll find the larger Recapture Reservoir and the nearby Red Cliffs and Anasazi ruins. Refer to resources at the Monticello Ranger District to learn more about all the recreational opportunities in the Abajos (**www.fs.fed.us/r4/ mantilasal/contact/monticello.shtml**).

Make sure you get up early in the morning before sunrise and take the drive toward Canyonlands National Park. Turn left out of the campground and drive west past Monticello Lake. After turning right at the fork, you'll begin your descent off the mountain. After only a few miles, you'll round bends in the road with astonishing views of the Needles district of Canyonlands. Layered red rock canyons, each more distant than the last, weave together to create a dramatic sandstone skyline. At sunrise, watch the top of each of these layered canyons come to life with light and then slowly become illuminated down to their base. Pull over at any of the graded turnouts to take it all in. Come prepared with extra batteries for your camera—you may need them.

There are opportunities to hike in the Abajo Mountains, but you'll have to search to find them. Though more typically known for its horse trails, this area can offer some surprises for hikers who are willing to work. For an easy-to-find trail that takes you to the 11,362-foot Abajo Peak, turn left out of the campground and go about a half mile to Forest Service Road 079, also known as North Canyon Road; it's on the left side of the road. Park here and begin your ascent toward the peak. After about 3 miles, you can leave the road on a faint footpath, or continue on the more established route. Once you summit, you'll be rewarded with views of the mountains and surrounding colorful canyons.

Dalton Springs is a practical alternative if you're visiting Canyonlands. Campgrounds near the park are scorching hot in the summer, and the Abajos provide a welcome respite from the sun. If you don't mind a beautiful 45-minute drive that meanders through

KEY INFORMATION

ADDRESS:	Manti-La Sal National Forest Monticello Ranger District 496 East Central Monticello, UT 84535
OPERATED BY:	United Land Management
INFORMATION:	www.publiclands .org
OPEN:	May–October (water availability varies)
SITES:	16
EACH SITE HAS:	Picnic table, metal fire ring
ASSIGNMENT:	First come, first served; no reservation
REGISTRATION:	Self-register on-site
FACILITIES:	Vault toilets, water spigots, garbage service
PARKING:	At campsites only
FEE:	$8 per night ($4 when water is unavailable); $12 for double sites (1 and 14)
ELEVATION:	8,402 feet
RESTRICTION:	*Pets:* Leashed *Fires:* In rings only *Other:* No saddle or pack animals

MAP

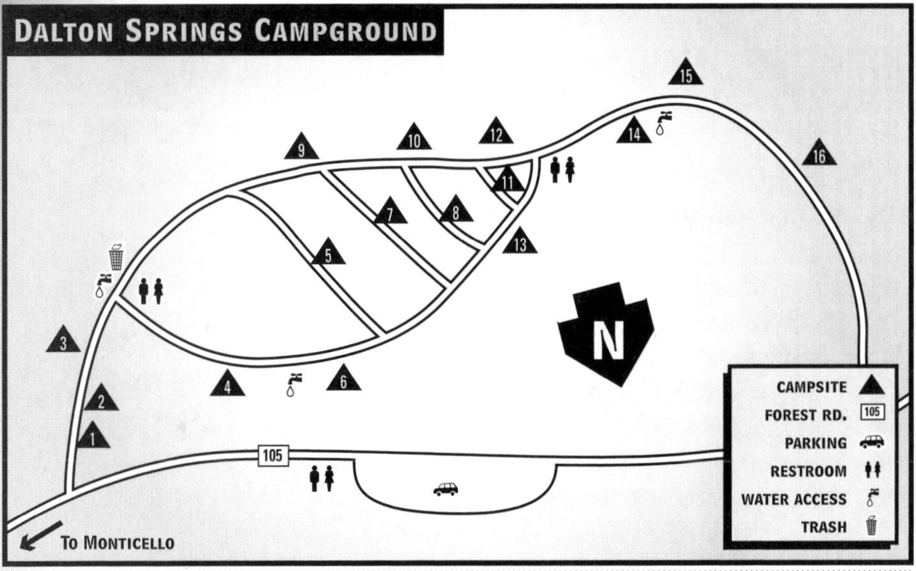
DALTON SPRINGS CAMPGROUND
1
2
3
4
5
6
7
8
9
10
11
12
13
14
15
16
N
105
TO MONTICELLO
CAMPSITE
FOREST RD.
105
PARKING
RESTROOM
WATER ACCESS
TRASH

GETTING THERE

From Interstate 70, take exit 182 onto US 191 South. Drive 86 miles to Monticello. Turn right on 200 South (FS 105) and drive 6 miles on paved road to the campground.

juniper and then aspens and pines, stay above the heat and chaos by choosing Dalton Springs as your base camp.

The Abajo Mountains are a welcome sight to wary winter eyes. To find out for sure when Dalton Springs Campground will open this spring, call the Monticello Ranger District at (435) 587-2041.

GPS COORDINATES

UTM Zone:12
Easting:637824
Northing:4192983
Latitude: N 37.87391
Longitude: W 109.43293

48
MOONFLOWER CAMPGROUND

I **F ADVENTURE HAS A HOME ADDRESS,** you can bet it's got a Moab zip code. This small town of 5,000 is the hub of activity in southeastern Utah. It's the headquarters of mountain biking, hiking, river running, and four-wheel drive exploration. Main Street Moab is like the Las Vegas Strip for outdoor enthusiasts (addicts), with dozens of guides, outfitters, and gear rental shops. It's high-octane adventure within easy reach of high-calorie fast-food joints.

It's no wonder thousands of people flock to this town each year. It's an exciting place to be, but the constant buzz of activity can make you dizzy. How great it is then, to have a place like the campground at Moonflower Canyon to dull out the noise and recharge your batteries overnight for the next day's adventure.

Moonflower is a magical place. It's only 3 miles from Moab, but seems like 300. While Moab moves at a frantic pace, Moonflower remains oblivious. The campground follows a small and narrow canyon that begins at a parking area along Kane Creek Road. The massive sheer walls wrap around a small trail dotted with eight walk-in campsites within the Behind the Rocks Wilderness Study Area. As you move deeper into the canyon, the noises of the busy road fade away and you're left with only silence in the cool air of the shaded campground.

There's no doubt that site 6 is the jewel of Moonflower. Set far away from the other sites, you'll feel like you're in the middle of nowhere as your tent is set underneath the trees and nestled against the canyon wall. Sites 4 through 8 are also nice, but just a bit closer together than the ideal. I'd recommend staying away from sites 1 through 3 unless you're a heavy sleeper. Kane Creek Road always has plenty of traffic and the engine sounds still reach these sites and bounce off the canyon walls.

> *Moonflower is a magical place. It's only 3 miles from Moab, but seems like 300.*

RATINGS

Beauty: ✪ ✪ ✪ ✪
Privacy: ✪ ✪ ✪ ✪
Spaciousness: ✪ ✪ ✪
Quiet: ✪ ✪ ✪ ✪
Security: ✪ ✪ ✪ ✪
Cleanliness: ✪ ✪ ✪ ✪ ✪

ADDRESS: Bureau of Land
Management
Moab Field Office
82 East Dogwood
Moab, UT 84532

OPERATED BY: Bureau of Land
Management
Moab Field Office

INFORMATION: www.blm.gov/utah/
moab

OPEN: Year-round

SITES: 8

EACH SITE HAS: Metal fire ring

ASSIGNMENT: First come,
first served; no
reservation

REGISTRATION: Self-register on-site

FACILITIES: Vault toilets,
garbage service

PARKING: 2 vehicles per site,
at campsites only

FEE: $10 per night

ELEVATION: 5,842 feet

RESTRICTION: *Pets:* Leashed
Fires: In rings only
Other: 2 vehicles,
2 tents, 6 people per
site

There are campgrounds all along Kane Creek Road, but the pavement ends a few miles after Moonflower. Although I saw a hardy family sedan make it down to the Echo Campground, I'd feel more comfortable in something with four-wheel drive or at least a higher ground clearance. The dirt road may also become impassable in the rain. Shortly after Echo, you'll leave the Colorado River to follow Kane Springs Creek. You'll pass over a cattle guard flanked on the right by a large boulder, and from there dispersed camping is common. There are many mountain bike, hiking, and Jeep trail options.

The best way to start your own adventure in Moab is to visit the city's information center, conveniently located on the southeast corner of Main and Center Streets in Moab. Here you'll find stands of free brochures ranging from public land information to the obligatory "Please spend your money with us!" promotional materials. Ask the knowledgeable staff and they'll help you narrow down your choices to find the option that best suits you. There's also a small bookstore and gift shop. As you know, a great guidebook is an invaluable tool when planning your valuable vacation days.

Just 5 miles farther up Kane Creek Road from Moonflower Canyon is Hunters Canyon. From a small parking area here you can begin your exploration of this rugged canyon. Hunter Arch is a popular hiking destination. Although the arch itself isn't the biggest or most spectacular arch in the area, the hike through Navajo Sandstone is enjoyable and the destination notable.

One of the most popular activities for visitors to Moab is river rafting. The Colorado River can accommodate paddlers of all abilities, from kids to hard-core kayakers. There's no shortage of river guides, but tours can fill up quickly so it's best to book ahead. You can visit the Moab Information Center online at **www.discovermoab.com** for more information about local guides and outfitters.

Moab is world-renowned for its mountain biking. The most talked-about trail in town is the Slickrock Trail, and with good reason. This 10.5-mile loop trail over sandstone opens up at its peak to reveal a staggering view of the Colorado River. It can be a rough trail

MAP

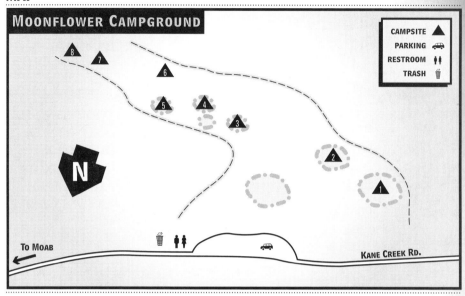

MOONFLOWER CAMPGROUND

CAMPSITE ▲
PARKING 🚐
RESTROOM ♦♦
TRASH 🗑

N

To Moab

Kane Creek Rd.

in parts, requiring riders to be in good physical shape. If you're a little rusty (or if your bike is, for that matter), you may want to take the 2-mile practice loop before heading out on the actual trail. To get to the Slickrock trail, go east on 300 South in Moab. Turn right when the road ends, then take your second left. You'll enter the Sand Flats Recreation Area where you'll have to pay a $5 fee, then go about a half mile to the trailhead.

When you come to Moab, bring your sense of adventure and plenty of ibuprofen. There are more adventures here than you could fulfill in a lifetime, and no better place to start them than from the quiet and magical Moonflower Campground.

GETTING THERE

From Interstate 70, take Exit 182 onto US 191 South and drive 31 miles south to Moab. In Moab, continue south to the traffic light at Kane Road. Turn right and drive 3 miles to the campground.

GPS COORDINATES

UTM Zone:12
Easting:623114
Northing:4268253
Latitude: N 38.55419
Longitude: W 109.58708

49
WARNER LAKE CAMPGROUND

> *This 21-site campground is the perfect place to seek refuge from the sizzling sun.*

THE COMBINATION OF HIGH MOUNTAIN peaks and cool summer temperatures is a rare and special treat in southeastern Utah, but that's exactly what you'll find at Warner Lake Campground. An often overlooked alternative to campgrounds down in the valley below, Warner Lake is close to Moab and both Arches and Canyonlands National Parks (around 45 minutes to Arches, a little more than an hour to Canyonlands).

Stay in the Manti-La Sal National Forest at Warner Lake and you'll be in a completely different world than the tens of thousands of tenting tourists who visit southeastern Utah each year. This 21-site campground is the perfect place to seek refuge from the sizzling sun that beats down on the baked sandstone and dusty roads of the river valley.

Don't think that the La Sal mountains are just an out-of-the way stop for national park experiences, though. The small pocket of mountains in this region can holds its own as a recreational destination. Hiking, biking, fishing, and scenic drives make the La Sals a unique and rewarding place.

Make certain to drive to the north side of the mountains to enjoy incredible views of the Colorado River valley and the many rock spires that line the sheer canyon walls. Take the La Sal Loop Road north for about 15 miles. As the road curves east you'll begin to descend and a scene deserving of your camera's panoramic mode will unfold in front of you.

In early spring you'll be treated to an abundant population of butterflies. The flits of blue, orange, and black wings dart in and out of your sight and accompany you as you stroll through the campground. Deer are also common in this area. On my visit I watched a group of five does mosey right through the middle of

RATINGS

Beauty: ☆ ☆ ☆ ☆ ☆
Privacy: ☆ ☆ ☆
Spaciousness: ☆ ☆ ☆
Quiet: ☆ ☆ ☆
Security: ☆ ☆
Cleanliness: ☆ ☆ ☆ ☆

the campground. I wondered if they had made a reservation.

Fishing at Warner Lake, a small reservoir, can be fast for small rainbow trout. Rainbows are usually planted around the beginning of June and again in July each year and make for a relaxing way to pass an afternoon.

Hiking trails are plentiful in this mountain range, and Warner Lake is the jumping-off point for many of the best. Take the trail to Oohwah Lake. It begins just past the fence at the far end of Warner Lake. Although you can drive to Oohwah by backtracking on La Sal Loop Road and taking the 3-mile dirt road at the Oohwah Campground turnoff, you'd miss the dynamic views of the aspen and pine tree line as it gradually turns to juniper and then red sandstone cliffs. Be prepared to huff and puff on the hike back because you'll have to come back up nearly 800 feet over the 1.5-mile trail, and it's *all* uphill. If you have multiple drivers in your group, you can send someone at Oohwah to shuttle hikers back to camp.

At Oohwah, you'll enjoy a typical alpine lake also stocked with small rainbows for fishing. Oohwah is home to a small campground, which is less developed but may be an alternative if Warner Lake is full. You'll also find a trailhead for the Clark Lake hike, which is just a short jaunt up the creek from Oohwah.

From Warner Lake you can also choose from trails to other destinations with dramatic views: Miners Basin at 2 miles, Burro Pass at 4 miles, and the Dry Fork-Beaver Basin Trail at 5 miles.

Warner Lake is popular on weekends, so make your reservations far in advance. For maximum privacy, try sites 5, 7, 10, and 11. Each is set back a bit from the road and somewhat shielded by thick aspen trunks. If you'd like more space, sites 14 and 16 back up into an open field and present unobstructed views of Haystack Mountain. Despite the fact that the campground also rents a small cabin and accommodates some larger RVs, it receives a healthy mix of tents and trailers and has a leisurely vibe.

Autumn is also busier than you might expect. The leaves in the La Sal Mountains ignite in color when the

KEY INFORMATION

ADDRESS:	Manti-La Sal National Forest Moab Ranger District 2290 South West Resource Boulevard Moab, UT 84532
OPERATED BY:	United Land Management
INFORMATION:	www.publiclands .org
OPEN:	May–October (water availability varies)
SITES:	21
EACH SITE HAS:	Picnic table, metal fire ring
ASSIGNMENT:	By reservation; first come, first served if available
REGISTRATION:	Online at www .reservusa.com or call (877) 444-6777
FACILITIES:	Vault toilets, water spigots
PARKING:	At campsites only; day parking available
FEE:	$10 per night ($5 when water is unavailable)
ELEVATION:	9,411 feet
RESTRICTION:	*Pets:* Leashed *Fires:* In rings only

MAP

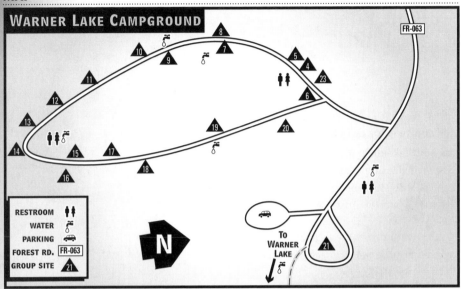

WARNER LAKE CAMPGROUND FR-063

RESTROOM	🚻
WATER	
PARKING	🚗
FOREST RD.	FR-063
GROUP SITE	🔺21

N

To
WARNER
LAKE

GETTING THERE

From Interstate 70, take exit 182 onto US 191 South. Drive approximately 37 miles to the signed La Sal Loop Road turn (just past mile marker 118). Turn left on La Sal Loop Road and drive for 16 miles to the signed campground turnoff. Turn right and drive 4 miles on a graded dirt road to the campground.

GPS COORDINATES

UTM Zone:12
Easting:650252
Northing:4264969
Latitude: N 38.52044
Longitude: W 109.27646

season begins to change. The radiant yellow leaves of the aspens look like paint strokes on the canvas of the canyon slopes. This spectacular show is idyllic for any fall-loving photographer.

Lock your car and secure your belongings, just to be safe. While the campground is more remote and up a dirt road, the area attracts day visitors and has a large group camping area. Locks will help honest people stay that way.

If you can only get away to Canyonlands and Arches National Parks during the summer, book a site at Warner Lake and beat the heat. It's worth the extra drive time to sleep sweatless. But don't overlook the La Sals and their own distinctive charm. There's plenty here to keep you busy and make your camping trip a memorable one.

50
GOBLIN VALLEY
STATE PARK

IMAGINE A PLACE WHERE little stone creatures dot the landscape like an eclectic mix of squatty snowmen, magical mushrooms, and tiny huts. Sounds pretty bizarre, right? I don't think they'll be putting "bizarre" on their brochure anytime soon, but that's definitely one way to describe Goblin Valley State Park.

These strange stone formations, commonly referred to as hoodoos, are actually made of eroded Entrada sandstone—worn from former highlands and deposited on the flat valley floor. The alternating layers of sandstone, siltstone, and shale now remain in the form of fantastic rock formations that seem to bubble up from the earth, like warts on the desert landscape.

The campground here in the valley of hoodoos has recently been renovated into a top-notch facility. The ranger station, once referred to as their "outhouse," is now a small visitor center. Old restrooms and portable toilets have given way to modern flush toilets and shower facilities. Each campsite has its own shade pavilion. The upside to all of this is that staying at Goblin Valley is more comfortable than ever; the downside is that more and more people are visiting, which makes camping cramped.

Goblin Valley Campground is a single loop with some sites spurred individually and others sharing a common parking area. The campground is clean and very well maintained, but sites are squished together and privacy is at a minimum. If at all possible, try for sites 12 or 19. Site 12 allows you to tuck your tent behind a rock wall and shield yourself from your neighbors, and site 19 is all by itself at the last corner of the campground loop. The sites are also on the smallish side, though the shade pavilion and picnic table provide enough space for you to set out the essentials.

> *Goblin Valley excites the mind and enlivens the imagination with images of oddly shaped desert hoodoos.*

RATINGS

Beauty: ✰ ✰ ✰ ✰
Privacy: ✰
Spaciousness: ✰ ✰
Quiet: ✰ ✰ ✰
Security: ✰ ✰ ✰
Cleanliness: ✰ ✰ ✰ ✰ ✰

KEY INFORMATION

ADDRESS: Goblin Valley State Park
P.O. Box 637
Green River, UT
84525-0637

OPERATED BY: Utah State Parks and Recreation

INFORMATION: www.stateparks.utah.gov

OPEN: Year-round

SITES: 24

EACH SITE HAS: Picnic table, shade covering, fire ring

ASSIGNMENT: By reservation; first come, first served if available

REGISTRATION: Call (800) 322-3770 or register at park entrance

FACILITIES: Visitor center, flush toilets, showers, drinking water

PARKING: 2 vehicles per site

FEE: $15 per night single use; $75 minimum group use; $6 park entrance

ELEVATION: 5,200 feet

RESTRICTIONS: *Pets:* Leashed
Other: 14-day stay limit

Vegetation around the campground is sparse, but provides a good lesson in desert survival. The hardy plants that do eke out a life in the desert are well adapted to long dry spells and expend little energy to grow. Look around for Mormon Tea (an ephedra plant), Russian thistle, Indian ricegrass, and different species of cacti.

Spring and fall are the best times to visit Goblin Valley. Summers are insufferably hot with little reprieve from the blazing sun. Temperatures often reach the low 100s, although at night they can fall to the mid 60s. Winter would also make a unique visit, as it has been known to snow within the park. Seeing little goblins with puffy white hats would be worth the inconvenience of a little desert mud and frigid nighttime temperatures.

Reservations are accepted March 15 through October 15, and are strongly recommended. The park was packed when I went on a Wednesday morning in April, so showing up for the weekend and getting a spot is unlikely. Due to its remote location, there aren't many other established campgrounds in the area, although dispersed camping is always an option.

Adjust to constantly seeing and being seen by your camping neighbors and you'll fall in love with the geology of Goblin Valley. Drive to the observation point southeast of the campground and you'll marvel at the hundreds of hoodoos below. An interpretive display explains in detail how the formations were created, and the wooden deck provides the perfect place to take pictures. Every so often a tour bus drops off visitors who descend on the valley floor, so take advantage of the convenience of your camp and get the coveted "people-less" photo. When the sun has nearly set, you'll get eerie pictures of the ghostlike shadows cast by the odd sandstone ogres.

If you'd rather set out on foot, the park offers three trails: Carmel Canyon, a 1.5-mile loop from the parking area to the desert floor; Curtis Bench, an easy 2.1-mile out-and-back trail along the Curtis formation; and Entrada Canyon, a 1.3-mile trail to the goblins from the campground. Each one offers a different perspective on the distinctive rock structures.

MAP

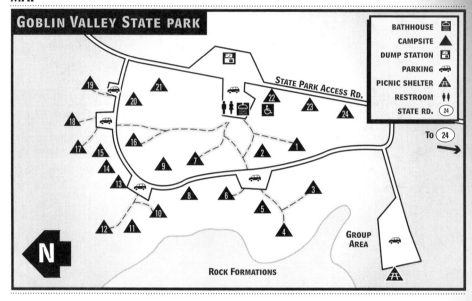

GOBLIN VALLEY STATE PARK

BATHHOUSE
CAMPSITE ▲
DUMP STATION
PARKING
PICNIC SHELTER
RESTROOM ††
STATE RD. ㉔

STATE PARK ACCESS RD.

To ㉔ →

N

ROCK FORMATIONS

GROUP AREA

Goblin Valley excites the mind and enlivens the imagination with images of oddly shaped desert hoodoos. They've been likened to mushrooms, warts, cottages, and chess pieces. What will you see on your visit?

GETTING THERE

Take Interstate 70 exit 149 (UT 24 West), located just west of Green River. Drive southwest nearly 30 miles to the well-marked park turnoff. Follow the paved road approximately 15 miles to the park.

GPS COORDINATES

UTM Zone: 12
Easting: 525058
Northing: 4269352
Latitude: N38.57227
Longitude: W110.71234

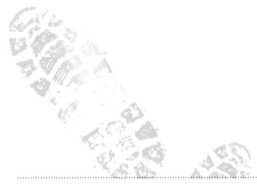

APPENDIXES **AND INDEX**

APPENDIX A:
CAMPING-EQUIPMENT
CHECKLIST

Except for the large and bulky items on this list, we keep a plastic storage container full of the essentials for car camping, so they're ready to go when we are. We make a last-minute check of the inventory, resupply anything that's low or missing, and away we go.

COOKING UTENSILS
Bottle opener
Bottles of salt, pepper, spices, sugar, cooking oil, and maple syrup in waterproof, spill-proof containers
Can opener
Cups, plastic or tin
Dish soap (biodegradable), sponge, and towel
Flatware
Food of your choice
Frying pan
Fuel for stove
Matches in waterproof container
Plates
Pocketknife
Pot with lid
Spatula
Stove
Tin foil
Wooden spoon

FIRST AID KIT
Band-Aids
First aid cream
Gauze pads
Ibuprofen or aspirin
Insect repellent
Moleskin
Snakebite kit
Sunscreen/chapstick
Tape, waterproof adhesive

SLEEPING GEAR
Pillow
Sleeping bag
Sleeping pad, inflatable or insulated
Tent with ground tarp and rainfly

MISCELLANEOUS
Bath soap (biodegradable), washcloth, and towel
Camp chair
Candles
Cooler
Deck of cards
Fire starter
Flashlight with fresh batteries
Foul weather clothing
Maps (road, topographic, trails, etc.)
Paper towels
Plastic zip-top bags
Sunglasses
Toilet paper
Water bottle
Wool blanket

OPTIONAL
Barbecue grill
Binoculars
Books on bird, plant, and wildlife identification
Cell phone
Fishing rod and tackle
GPS
Hatchet
Lantern

APPENDIX B:
SOURCES OF INFORMATION

ASHLEY NATIONAL FOREST
355 North Vernal Avenue
Vernal, UT 84078
(435) 789-1181
www.fs.fed.us/r4/ashley

DIXIE NATIONAL FOREST
1789 North Wedgewood Lane
Cedar City, UT 84720
(435) 865-3700
www.fs.fed.us/r4/dixie

FISHLAKE NATIONAL FOREST
115 East 900 North
Richfield, UT 84701
(435) 896-9233
www.fs.fed.us/r4/fishlake

MANTI-LA SAL NATIONAL FOREST
599 West Price River Drive
Price, UT 84501
(435) 637-2817
www.fs.fed.us/r4/mantilasal

SAWTOOTH NATIONAL FOREST
2647 Kimberly Road East
Twin Falls, ID 83301
(208) 737-3200
www.fs.fed.us/r4/sawtooth

UINTA NATIONAL FOREST
88 West 100 North
P.O. Box 1428
Provo, UT 84601
(801) 342-5100
www.fs.fed.us/r4/uinta

WASATCH-CACHE NATIONAL FOREST
125 South State Street
Salt Lake City, UT 84138
(801) 236-3400
www.fs.fed.us/r4/wcnf

BUREAU OF LAND MANAGEMENT
440 West 200 South, Suite 500
Salt Lake City, UT 84101
(801) 539-4001
www.ut.blm.gov

UTAH STATE PARKS
1594 West North Temple
Salt Lake City, UT 84116
(801) 538-7220
www.stateparks.utah.gov

PUBLIC LANDS INFORMATION CENTER
www.publiclands.org

TOPOZONE
(online topographical maps)
www.topozone.com

UTAH DIVISION OF WILDLIFE RESOURCES
1594 West North Temple
Salt Lake City, UT 84116
(801) 538-4700
www.wildlife.utah.gov

ZION NATIONAL PARK
Springdale, UT 84767
(435) 772-3256
www.nps.gov/zion

APPENDIX B
SOURCES OF
INFORMATION (CONTINUED)

BRYCE CANYON NATIONAL PARK
P.O. Box 640201
Bryce Canyon, UT 84764-0201
(435) 834-5322
www.nps.gov/brca

CAPITOL REEF NATIONAL PARK
HC 70 Box 15
Torrey, UT 84775
(435) 425-3791 ext. 111
www.nps.gov/care

CANYONLANDS NATIONAL PARK
2282 SW Resource Boulevard
Moab, UT 84532
(435) 719-2313
www.nps.gov/cany

ARCHES NATIONAL PARK
P.O. Box 907
Moab, UT 84532
(435) 719-2299
www.nps.gov/arch

NATURAL BRIDGES NATIONAL MONUMENT
HC 60 Box 1
Lake Powell, UT 84533
(435) 692-1234
www.nps.gov/nabr

INDEX

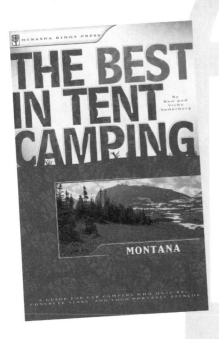

BEST IN TENT CAMPING: MONTANA

by Ken and Vicky Soderberg
ISBN 10: 0-89732-598-2
ISBN 13: 978-0-89732-598-1
$14.95
192 pages

Montana is a paradise for outdoor lovers, especially tent campers. Ken and Vicky Soderberg traveled throughout the state and selected the 50 most beautiful campgrounds for **The Best in Tent Camping: Montana**, ensuring a wonderful location whether going on an overnight trip or a weeklong vacation.

GPS OUTDOORS

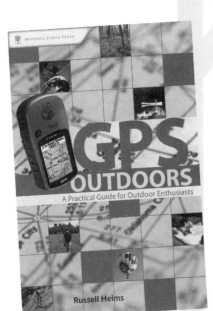

by Russell Helms
ISBN 10: 0-89732-967-8
ISBN 13: 978-0-89732-967-5
$10.95
120pages

Whether you're a hiker on a weekend trip through the Great Smokies, a backpacker cruising the Continental Divide Trail, a mountain biker kicking up dust in Moab, a paddler running the Lewis and Clark bicentennial route, or a climber pre-scouting the routes up Mount Shasta, a simple handheld GPS unit is fun, useful, and can even be a lifesaver.

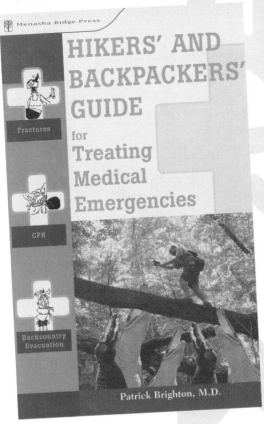

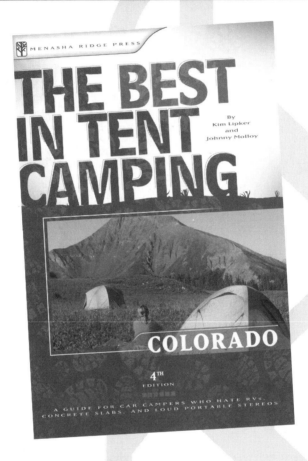

DEAR CUSTOMERS AND FRIENDS,

SUPPORTING YOUR INTEREST IN OUTDOOR ADVENTURE, travel, and an active lifestyle is central to our operations, from the authors we choose to the locations we detail to the way we design our books. Menasha Ridge Press was incorporated in 1982 by a group of veteran outdoorsmen and professional outfitters. For 25 years now, we've specialized in creating books that benefit the outdoors enthusiast.

Almost immediately, Menasha Ridge Press earned a reputation for revolutionizing outdoors- and travel-guidebook publishing. For such activities as canoeing, kayaking, hiking, backpacking, and mountain biking, we established new standards of quality that transformed the whole genre, resulting in outdoor-recreation guides of great sophistication and solid content. Menasha Ridge continues to be outdoor publishing's greatest innovator.

The folks at Menasha Ridge Press are as at home on a white-water river or mountain trail as they are editing a manuscript. The books we build for you are the best they can be, because we're responding to your needs. Plus, we use and depend on them ourselves.

We look forward to seeing you on the river or the trail. If you'd like to contact us directly, join in at www.trekalong.com or visit us at www.menasharidge.com. We thank you for your interest in our books and the natural world around us all.

SAFE TRAVELS,

Bob Sehlinger

BOB SEHLINGER
PUBLISHER

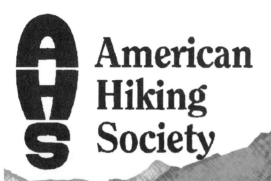
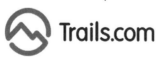
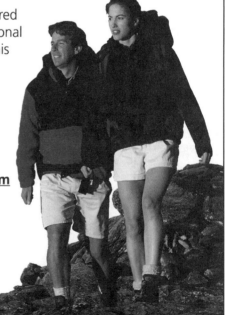